Choosing Unsafe Sex

Choosing Unsafe Sex

AIDS-Risk Denial Among
Disadvantaged Women

Elisa J. Sobo

University of Pennsylvania Press

Philadelphia

Contents

Preface

In this book, I describe the findings from an anthropological study of the links between inner-city women's condom use rates and their experiences and understandings of heterosexual relationships. I also discuss findings from a smaller project on seropositivity self-disclosure among HIV-positive individuals.

The condom use research took place in Cleveland, Ohio, over a two-year period between 1991 and 1993. I began the study at the request of Dr. Philip Toltzis, who oversees health education for women seeking pregnancy-related care at the five urban health care centers associated with Cleveland's Maternity and Infant Health Care Program (M&I). Alarmed by the rising rates of HIV infections and AIDS among the poor, urban, mostly Black women who use the M&I clinics, Toltzis directed staff members to include AIDS and safer sex information in their educational efforts. But according to clinic records and staff reports clients did not comply with the pro-condom advice they were given.

Toltzis assumed that the clients were not stupid and that their non-use of condoms was not a result of ignorance of the facts about HIV transmission. The clients were well-informed of these facts by clinic staff members. But, as Toltzis also knew, sometimes health education messages do not make an impact because of communication problems — sometimes "doctor's orders" simply do not make sense to the people being asked to comply with them. Toltzis guessed that cultural barriers were probably blocking full communication between his AIDS educators and their clients, and he saw that an anthropological approach to AIDS education could help. So, from his office in the Pediatrics and Infectious Disease division at Rainbow Babies' and Children's Hospital, Toltzis rang up Dr. Jill Korbin, an anthropologist at Case Western Reserve University who shared his interest in urban pediatric health. Toltzis hoped that Korbin could help him out.

About that time, I arrived at Case Western Reserve's anthropology department, where I would be working as a postdoctoral research fellow. I had recently completed a book concerning the links between traditional health beliefs and sexuality, procreation, contraception, and gender relations in Jamaica (Sobo 1993). While I planned to continue analyzing data from the Jamaican research during my time at Case Western Reserve, I also wanted to involve myself in research locally. Korbin knew that I was interested in reproductive health issues and suggested I meet with Toltzis to discuss his needs. After a long discussion with Toltzis about the program and its problems, I agreed to design and carry out a research project. Toltzis secured some seed money for research and I began to plan.

Data collection commenced in the fall of 1991 and concluded in the summer of 1993; it was carried out at the J. Glen Smith Health Clinic and at Bellflower House, one of Cleveland's social welfare centers. Grants from the Community AIDS Partnership Project and the Spring Foundation for Research on Contemporary Women supported the research. I conducted most of the final analyses in 1993 and 1994 at New Mexico State University (NMSU), where I was Assistant Professor of Anthropology. I initiated the seropositivity self-disclosure research with the aid of grants from NMSU and from the Southern Area Health Education Center/Border Health Education Training Center. The manuscript for this book was prepared at NMSU and revised at the University of California's Center for AIDS Prevention Studies in San Francisco, where Dr. Thomas Hall kindly invited me to work as a visiting scholar in the summer of 1994.

Clinicians and social workers who helped with the research include Donna Dayse, Ina Adkins, Barbara Hood, Linda Michael, Megan McGuire, David Simonsmeier, Carl Valles, Deborah Washington, Gail Wheeler, and Karen Young. Drs. Jill Korbin and Philip Toltzis were also instrumental. Margaret Ruble ably supervised the data collection for the first phase of the research in Cleveland, during which Sara Colegrove, Sandra Marchese, and Candis Platt helped us gather data. Jude Drapeau, Delia Easton, Joanna Skilogianis, and Maria Armstrong also helped with data collection at various points in the project. Michelle Nawrocki transcribed interview and focus group tapes. Timi Barone, Heather Lindstrom, Barbara Meek, Jennifer Rutkowski, and Joanna Skilogianis helped with quantitative data management and preliminary statistics; Dr. Richard Glaze provided enormous assistance with the final quantitative analyses. Samantha Coppa, Michelle Nawrocki, and Adina Sobo proofread the manuscript.

Colleagues who read and commented on various sections of the book (in their various manifestations) include Drs. Robert Carlson, Paul Farmer, Byron Good, Mary-Jo DelVecchio Good, Colleen Jonsson, Kay Kinsey, Jill Korbin, William Leap, Shirley Lindenbaum, Janet McGrath, Kathleen O'Connor, and Scott Rushforth. Anonymous reviewers also provided great assistance. Several sections of the book were adapted from articles published elsewhere, and I thank the editors and the anonymous reviewers from these journals for their constructive suggestions.

During the course of the research for this book, I also was engaged in a complementary project with homeless adolescents. My work on the latter project informed (as it was sometimes informed by) my work on the former. Funded by grants from Case Western Reserve's University Center for Adolescent Health (UCAH) and from the Armington Research Program on Values in Children, supported by UCAH Director Dr. Frederick Robbins, the teens project was carried out with co-investigator Dr. Gregory Zimet, UCAH Sexuality Subcommittee members Drs. Teena Zimmerman, JoAnn Jackson, Joan Mortimer, and Rina Lazebnik, and UCAH Associate Director Carlyn Yanda.

In addition to colleagues, various relatives and friends deserve mention. I am especially grateful to Lillian Mintz, Dr. Harvey Smallman, David and Naomi Sobo, and Dr. Elinor Velasquez for their encouragement. I am indebted to Deborah Shreve for her assistance in identifying a primary funding source for the research. I also wish to thank Ellyn Taylor for her support, and I owe many thanks to the Friedmans, the Haywoods, and the Schwartzes for the gracious hospitality that they extended to me during my stay in Cleveland.

The good will and assistance of all of the above-named individuals and funding agencies notwithstanding, I am most indebted to the people who participated as "subjects" in this project. These individuals contributed more than their time: they contributed their stories and they contributed parts of themselves, in a sense, to the fight against AIDS. Confidentiality and anonymity concerns bar me from mentioning all participants by name, but thanks are due to them nonetheless. Without them, this book would not exist.

Dental & the flow of
sexual information

Chapter 1
Introduction

The popular and scientific media often describe people who are at risk for human immunodeficiency virus (HIV) infection but fail to use condoms as being "in denial." Unfortunately, most authors, clinicians, and health officials — indeed, most people — take the specifics of the denial process for granted. Denial has become a blanket term in the most literal sense, tossed about freely, covering up or hiding away the broad range of complex factors that contribute to Acquired Immunodeficiency Syndrome (AIDS) risk misperceptions and unprotected (e.g., condomless penetrative-receptive) sex. Until we examine these factors and arrive at an understanding of the mechanisms of AIDS-risk denial, we will be unable to suggest effective ways to lessen the denial, and we will continue to be limited in our ability to decrease the high rates of unsafe sex it entails.

The research described in this book takes a critical approach to AIDS-risk denial, providing insight into how and why it occurs. Findings suggest that women who hold certain expectations for heterosexual unions actually *need* to practice unsafe sex in order to support their beliefs that their own unions meet these expectations. Women seem to have a related tendency to assume that they have themselves been tested for HIV sero-positivity (antibodies to the human immunodeficiency virus) when they have not. Both unsafe sexual practice and the tendency to assume testing stem from wishful thinking engendered by women's hopes for their relationships and their desires to preserve status and self-esteem.

AIDS is on the rise among women — especially among poor Black and Latina inner-city women. Regular condom use can help stop the spread of HIV, but public response to warnings about the consequences of unprotected or unsafe (condomless) penetrative-receptive sex has not been enthusiastic. Most of us do not see ourselves as people at risk for AIDS. Few of us use condoms on a regular basis even though having condomless penetrative-receptive sex with an HIV-positive partner could lead to HIV infection. In the following chapters, I ask how and why we fail to acknowledge our own risk behaviors. I examine the mechanisms of heterosexual female AIDS-risk denial by exploring the reasons behind condom use rates and by investigating the cultural meanings and social ramifications that condom use and AIDS carry. I focus in particular on the condom-related practices and understandings of impoverished Black inner-city women.

Most of the data discussed in this book were collected at the instigation of Dr. Philip Toltzis, who directs and oversees health education for women seeking pregnancy-related care at the five urban health care centers associated with Cleveland's Maternity and Infant Health Care Program (M&I). Distressed by the rising rate of HIV infection among the poor inner-city minority women who use the M&I clinics, Dr. Toltzis asked me to design and carry out an anthropological study with clinic clients.

The goal for the project was to identify and qualitatively explore enablers of and barriers to safer-sex behavior among the clinic clients. What factors made it easier for women to get their male sex partners to use condoms? Were certain groups of women more likely than others to forgo condoms? If so, why? What were the differences between users and non-users? Figuring that actions which have costs also can have benefits, I elicited, described, and analyzed participants' perceptions of the social, economic, emotional, and other benefits of unsafe sex. I also explored women's perceptions of risk, power, and persecution, their social and economic situations, and their health-related cultural knowledge and explanatory models or ideas about AIDS and HIV infection.

The project was designed expressly for collecting data to be used in adjusting the M&I AIDS education curriculum to make it more effective. M&I records from 1991 showed that 90 percent of clients were impoverished and that 25 percent had some history of substance use (which, as defined by M&I, includes the use of alcohol as well as crack cocaine, heroin, or other drugs). About one-fourth of the clients were first-time mothers, and almost all clients had some characteristics—nutritional deficits, income limitations, drug habits—placing them in the "at risk" category.[1] Such information is important, because it gives us some ideas about clients' objective situations, but it reveals nothing about clients' subjective understandings of personal life experiences. It reveals nothing about their sex-related, condom-related, or AIDS-related beliefs and attitudes, nor does it tell us about the culture that encourages these beliefs and attitudes.

In the course of the research, I found that most of the participants usually chose to forgo condoms. They did so because they did not think that they could "catch AIDS." Most participants believed, as do most U.S.

adults (Schoenborn et al. 1994), that they were simply not at risk for AIDS. Most said that AIDS is a disease that only other people get.

The strength of participants' AIDS-risk denial intrigued me. It became a prominent issue in the research because of its power to inhibit the desire or perceived need for condoms: if we do not think that we are at risk, we are not likely to take precautions. In the end, I was able to isolate some of the major causes, contexts, and mechanisms of AIDS-risk denial. As I shall explain, this denial is linked to psychosocial well-being in ways that both enable and necessitate unsafe sex.

While the Cleveland research involved poor urban women, I do not believe that the denial complex I describe is limited to the urban Midwestern poor. Indeed, one of the factors that makes this AIDS-risk denial complex so interesting to me is its apparent pervasiveness. For instance, supplementary data from research carried out with HIV-positive individuals in the Southwest (described after the Cleveland data) indicate that this denial complex is at work there, too. Moreover, denial among the untested and the seronegative makes it very difficult for seropositive individuals to institute safer sex; they often find that partners and potential partners refuse to use condoms because they do not see the need for such protection.

The Cleveland study participants were not the only untested or apparently seronegative women who, over the course of the past few years, have assured me that they are not at risk for AIDS. Many of the narratives or stories told by participants could well have been told by my students, kindred, colleagues, and friends — generally relatively affluent people in comparison to the participants, and generally light-skinned and well-educated. Very little research on AIDS-risk denial involves affluent white suburban women, and I certainly do not wish to represent my casual observations among such women as conclusive. Nonetheless, if my suspicion regarding the pervasiveness of AIDS-risk denial is correct, the implications of these findings reach far beyond Cleveland's inner-city limits.

The findings reported here were submitted for use to Dr. Toltzis and the clinic staff in Cleveland. They also can be used by health educators in other predominantly Black urban neighborhoods to improve their own AIDS education programs. If I am correct in arguing that the denial complex I describe is related to mainstream U.S. gender and conjugal expectations, the findings can help educators working in other contexts as well. Furthermore, they can be used by those of us who want to gain a deeper understanding of our own assumptions about relationships and about our own sexual motives and unsafe habits. I hope these findings can help us to instigate the kinds of attitudinal and behavioral changes that so many of us have been uninterested in or reluctant to make.

The Structure of This Book

The present chapter provides an overview of the research and the book. Chapter 2 reviews some of the basic facts about AIDS and HIV, focusing on U.S. women, among whom AIDS and HIV infection rates are increasing disproportionately and swiftly. In 1992, the number of women with AIDS was 9.8 percent higher than in 1991. This rate of increase was almost four times than that for men (2.5%) during the same period (JAMA 1993). By the end of 1993, women represented about 12½ percent of the cumulative adult and adolescent AIDS cases reported (CDC 1994a). AIDS is the sixth leading cause of death among all U.S. women aged twenty-five to forty-four; it is the first leading cause of death in certain regions for women in this age group who live in urban poverty (CDC 1993a). Black women are overrepresented among the urban poor. They are also about sixteen times more likely than white women to be diagnosed with AIDS (CDC National AIDS Clearinghouse 1995). In anticipation of the research findings in later chapters, Chapter 2 provides some background information about Black sexual culture.

Chapter 3 explores past approaches to AIDS prevention, focusing on risk perception. Common sense tells us that public AIDS education programs are the key to increasing condom use. But interventions that focus on the didactic dissemination of factual information do not work, largely because members of the targeted populations do not personalize or apply to themselves the AIDS-related information provided to them. Chapter 3 explains the importance of culturally appropriate and gender sensitive approaches to AIDS education, and shows why methods of encouraging risk personalization are key to an approach's success.

Health education specialists have identified risk perception as one of the primary factors affecting health-related behavioral change. Self-esteem concerns and cognitive errors lead people to make optimistically biased evaluations of their chances for experiencing particular health problems. The perceived preventability of AIDS and its negative connotations increase people's tendency to view their own level of risk for it as minimal. People can also be optimistically biased in their evaluations of entire groups' risk for AIDS. The defensive function of this bias and of conspiracy and persecution rhetoric, such as discourse concerning CIA genocide plots, is addressed. Chapter 3 makes clear the impact of both macro- and micro-level psychocultural, social, political, and economic factors on people's risk reduction efforts.

Chapter 4 examines HIV seropositivity self-disclosure. Many people have heard or read anecdotes in which vindictive seropositive individuals spread HIV to unsuspecting others. These stories suggest that nothing one does to protect oneself from HIV infection will make the least bit of difference: whether or not condoms are used, rancorous seropositive individuals who want to spread HIV infection will find ways to do so. Furthermore, while many AIDS education programs stress the importance of "knowing" one's partner(s), these stories suggest that asking potential partners about their pasts is pointless: HIV-positive people will lie. Or will they? We actually know very little about the issues that seropositive people confront as they consider telling their lovers about their HIV infections. Chapter 4 reviews the data on this topic and suggests that the HIV scare story represents simply another *genre* of conspiratorial thought (albeit one that is unduly damaging to seropositive people).

Chapters 5 through 8 present material from the Cleveland study against the background of literature and theory already provided. Chapter 5 discusses the specific nature of the condom use research, describing the settings and methods, and supplementing quantitative demographic information regarding the participants with brief, qualitative biographical sketches and anecdotes. It explains the limitations of the study and discusses the kinds of generalizations supported by the findings. The research was conducted with a highly specific group of poor Black inner-city women and was not designed to produce generalizations regarding a broader segment of the population. But it and other AIDS prevention studies suggest that ethnicity is of limited causal significance; the main conclusions of the research are, I think, applicable to all women who share the participants' cultural beliefs about relationships. As Chapters 6, 7, and 8 show, these relationship beliefs are consistent with mainstream U.S. relationship ideals.

Most of the participants said that they did not rely on men for money; in light of this, Chapter 6 questions the assumption that men are breadwinners and that financial need leads women to capitulate to men's requirement that they forgo condoms. Women's views on financial dependence and independence are discussed, and their testimony about self-determination and their own sense of agency in relation to finances and in relation to the sexual arena is explored.

Chapters 7 and 8 examine the foundations and ramifications of optimistically biased perceptions of AIDS risk. Chapter 7 describes the psychosocial benefits of unsafe sex, which include enhanced self-esteem and status. In the absence of certain kinds of extraconjugal social support, and particularly in the presence of certain kinds of conjugal arrangements, cultural expectations for conjugal relationships lead women to practice unsafe sex; they also lead women to cast other men — but not their own partners — as likely to be unfaithful. Heterosexual relationship ideals, conjugal styles, and women's extraconjugal networks are examined, and condom-use patterns are evaluated in light of these factors.

Chapter 8 deals with HIV serostatus testing. It discusses the views participants, previous researchers, and officials hold on routine testing of at-risk women. It presents findings indicating that some women assume themselves to have been tested for HIV when in fact they have not and examines the wishful thinking, cognitive errors, and misinformation that can cause women to make this assumption.

Chapter 9 explores the impact of a positive test on attitudes toward relationships and sex. Findings from HIV seropositivity self-disclosure research indicate that seropositive people may frequently conceal their seropositivity, and that they may generally do so with good intentions rather than to inflict harm. With casual partners, HIV-positive people may prefer beneficent prophylaxis (nondisclosure accompanied by insistence on safer sex) to self-disclosure. When prophylactic action is refused by optimistically biased casual partners, seropositive individuals may abandon the idea of having sex, or they may interpret this lack of interest as the result of an informed choice and proceed with the intended sexual actions.

The final chapter, Chapter 10, sums up the findings and offers suggestions for improving interventions. Educators must not alienate targeted groups of women by insultingly suggesting that their male lovers are all unfaithful; rather, they should use approaches sensitive to cultural expectations for relationships. I recommend approaches using social marketing techniques, and I identify directions for future research. I then clarify the salience of the Cleveland project's findings for all women who have similar expectations, and suggest non-threatening ways for women to acknowledge their risks and introduce condoms into the sexual arena.

I must here make a few terminological justifications and clarifications. First, because the line between legal and common-law marriage was in many ways insignificant in the context of this research, I often use the word "conjugal" in an inclusive fashion, subsuming paraconjugal or common-law relationships. Second and more important, while I argue that "denial" is an ill-defined and over-used term, I have chosen to retain it instead of adding to the mountain of social-scientific jargon that we already have to contend with by inventing another label. I do so because readers will be familiar with the term to begin with and because I intend to convince readers that denial is not as simple a phenomenon as it at first appears. I hope that by the end of the next few chapters readers will understand the complexity of denial and will appreciate the problems associated with the uncritical use of the term.

I also have chosen to use participants' preferred terminology wherever I can. The majority of the women who participated in the research prefer to identify themselves as "Black" rather than as "African American," so I use the term "Black" to designate African American ethnicity through-

out the book.[2] I also use participants' language preferences when referring to HIV and AIDS, both of which participants simply called "AIDS."
Except in places where it is absolutely inappropriate, I do too.

While I use participants' terms, all names mentioned are pseudonyms.
Quotes are verbatim; however, I have taken the liberty of altering oral
grammar where doing so increases the written clarity of participants'
statements without altering their meanings. Finally, I should note that the
terms "condom users" and "users," refer to women who can get their
male sexual partners to use condoms or who agree to use condoms with
these partners; those women who do not desire to have partners wear
condoms or who cannot convince partners to do so are referred to as
"non-users" throughout the book.

Notes

1. These figures were provided by M&I record keeper Anne Gulbranse. The "at
risk" category is M&I's.

2. People from many nations have dark skin and so are included in cross-
culturally informed references to "Blacks." In this book I use the latter term, as
did participants, to refer specifically to non-Hispanic African Americans. I use
participants' terminology in an effort to allow them to speak for themselves in-
asmuch as this is possible.

Chapter 2
Women and AIDS in the United States

As I write, the cumulative total number of reported AIDS cases in the United States hovers at about 400,000. By the end of 1993, about 61 percent of all individuals who had been diagnosed with AIDS since its biomedical identification were dead (CDC 1994a). AIDS is the third leading cause of death among U.S. men and women aged twenty-five to forty-four; it is the ninth leading cause overall (CDC 1993d).

Most of the people who are now suffering from AIDS were infected years ago with Human Immunodeficiency Virus (HIV), the virus associated with AIDS. Today, between 550,000 and 1,000,000 U.S. residents are HIV positive (infected). The higher estimate, itself a downward correction for a 1986 Public Health Service estimate that up to 1,500,000 individuals harbored the virus, was arrived at during a workshop in 1989 (CDC 1990), and will remain the "official" Centers for Disease Control and Prevention (CDC) figure until the results of a 1994 workshop are announced. The lower estimate comes from an analysis of the first three years of data collected in a six-year national household survey carried out between 1988 and 1994 under the auspices of the National Center for Health Statistics (NCHS). The survey, called the National Health and Nutrition Examination Survey, collects data on numerous health topics using blood tests and other techniques (McQuillan et al. 1994).

The NCHS finding, which is about half the official CDC estimate, suggested to many researchers that HIV infections — and so AIDS cases — are not increasing as quickly as experts originally thought they would. But others point out that the survey did not cover people who do not live in private households, so prisoners, the homeless, and people who were hospitalized at the time of the study — people who are generally at an increased risk for HIV infection — are not represented in the figure given. Geraldine McQuillan, who oversaw the HIV data collection and analyses, suggests that, had these people been included, the figure might have been 600,000 rather than 550,000 (personal communication). She also notes that the NCHS figure of 550,000 represents a mid-range point in a carefully calculated interval estimate, and points out that confidence limits were large enough so that the top margin of the interval or range hit the CDC one-million mark (see McQuillan et al. 1994).

When the results of the 1994 HIV prevalence workshop are made public, it is expected that the official CDC estimate will be lowered (Ron Wilson, NCHS, personal communication). For now, however, a best guess might place the number of HIV-positive individuals in the United States somewhere between the current CDC estimate and the NCHS figure. That is, perhaps about 750,000 U.S. residents, or just under one in three hundred and fifty, are infected with HIV. But because of the nature of the pandemic it is very hard to know for sure.

HIV-positive U.S. residents currently account for about 5 percent of the fifteen million individuals worldwide who, according to a report issued by the World Health Organization (WHO) in early 1994, are infected with HIV (one million of these infections are in children). U.S. AIDS cases represent only 13 percent of the three million people worldwide who have AIDS or have died from it (WHO 1994). This chapter briefly describes the pandemic that has caused so much death and suffering, focusing in particular on the effects that AIDS has on U.S. women's lives. (For an overview of the global situation for women, see De Bruyn 1992; Gupta and Weiss 1993; see also Mann et al. 1992.)

Heightened AIDS Risks

Social-Structural Factors: An Overview

History has shown that HIV is not a discriminating virus: one human body is as good as the next as long as there is an easy way to enter it. Once an individual has been infected and has seroconverted (become HIV positive), the virus slowly effects the collapse of the immune system, resulting in AIDS. Upon being diagnosed with AIDS, the average remaining life span for whites is between eighteen and twenty-four months; for Blacks it is six months (Lester and Saxxon 1988). This discrepancy suggests that, unless the inbuilt immune systems of Blacks are radically different from those of whites, which they do not appear to be, AIDS is more than just a biological event.

Biologically, all HIV wants is a warm human body in which to thrive and reproduce. So, conceptually at least, every human being is at risk for HIV infection and AIDS. Nonetheless, behavioral, environmental, and gender-linked factors mean that risk is distributed unevenly through the human species. As far as behaviors go, unprotected penetrative-receptive sex — whether anal or vaginal — is especially risky. Like risky behaviors, living in an area where HIV infection rates are high increases the likeli-hood of one's own infection, simply because the chances of one's sexual partner(s) being infected are that much higher. Because urban areas, where so many impoverished Black women live, have the highest con-centrations of people with HIV, Black women generally have higher than average chances of contracting AIDS. (The same holds true for poor inner-city women of other ethnicities.)

In the aforementioned NCHS study, McQuillan et al. (1994) found about four times as many Blacks as whites or others to be infected with HIV (Hispanics also were disproportionately infected). Inner cities have become breeding grounds for HIV largely because of contemporary power (and so resource, etc.) inequities stemming from historically prob-lematic class and race relations. Unequal power relations also persist between the genders, and these further heighten poor minority women's risk for AIDS.

Risks for Women: A Deeper Look

AIDS is the leading cause of death for women between the ages of twenty and forty in the major cities of the Americas, Western Europe, and sub-Saharan Africa (Chin 1989, as cited in Bezemer 1992). United Nations Development Program figures indicate that every day, around the world, 500 women die of AIDS and 3,000 more become infected (Rensberger 1993). Worldwide, perhaps 1,500,000 women have AIDS or have died of AIDS; perhaps 7,000,000 are currently infected with HIV.

The underreporting of AIDS cases among women notwithstanding, women account for half of all AIDS cases in much of sub-Saharan Africa and in parts of the Caribbean. While in the United States and many European nations, AIDS hit first and hardest among homosexual men, even in these nations the proportion of total AIDS cases reported among women is rising. For example, in Frankfurt, Germany, the percentage of HIV-infected patients who are women rose from 4 percent in 1984 to 25 percent in 1988 (Carovano 1991).

In the United States, the annual percentage of AIDS cases among women rose at a fairly steady pace, from 3 percent in 1981 (Rosen and Blank 1992) to almost 14 percent in 1992 (CDC 1993a). For the 1991–92 period, the rate of increase in female cases (9.8%) was almost four times that of male cases (2.5%) (JAMA 1993). By 1993, women comprised nearly 16 percent of the annual total (CDC 1994a; it must be noted that a portion of these cases would not have counted as AIDS cases under the pre-1993 CDC definition, discussed later in this chapter).

Worldwide, women are currently being infected with HIV three times as quickly as men (*AIDS Alert* 1993). And most women get AIDS from

men: heterosexual transmission accounts for 90 percent of all female
cases of AIDS worldwide (*AIDS Alert* 1993) and 35 percent of U.S. female cases (CDC 1994a). In the United States, heterosexual transmission
edged out intravenous drug use as the most common mode of female infection in 1992 (JAMA 1993; note that men who transmit HIV to women
seem to have been themselves most often infected through intravenous
drug use).

Heterosexual transmission to women does not just mean transmission
through vaginal intercourse. While much heterosexual intercourse is
genital, many heterosexual couples have anal sex. At least 10 percent of
U.S. women aged fifteen through sixty-four are reported to "engage with
some frequency in anal intercourse," and 39 percent of U.S. women have
had at least one experience of anal sex (Voeller 1990, 296).

Women are more vulnerable than men to heterosexually transmitted
HIV infection, because women involved in heterosexual intercourse are
generally on the receiving (receptive) end. As reception involves at least
minimal tissue trauma, receiving women are at a biologically higher risk
for infection than their penetrating partners. This is especially true when
force is used during sex or when sex is tempestuous, when damage to
vaginal or anal tissue is more likely. Oral contraceptive use, the use of
intrauterine devices, and vaginal or other reproductive tract infections
increase women's susceptibility to HIV, as do the physiological changes
that accompany menstruation (Bezemer 1992).

Teen-aged girls are in a particularly vulnerable position biologically
because their vaginal linings are not as thick as those of mature women.
Furthermore, they are vulnerable from a sociodemographic point of view
because they often have sex with older men — men who have had more
opportunity for acquiring HIV infection. Worldwide, 70 percent of all
new female infectees are between the ages of fifteen and twenty-five
(Rensberger 1993). In the United States, the annual number of women
aged twenty through twenty-nine years who acquired AIDS heterosexually has increased by almost 97 percent since 1988 (JAMA 1993).

Anal sex is as dangerous for teen-aged girls as it is for adult women.
Girls often have anal sex as a way of protecting their (vaginal) virginity,
because they find it pleasurable, or for both reasons (furthermore, sometimes coercion is involved). Of the young women participating in a study
of sexual practices in New York City, 26 percent had engaged in anal
intercourse (Rensberger 1993).

In the United States, at this point in the AIDS pandemic, women have a
higher chance of having sex with an infected person than men do, because there is a large pool of bisexual men (men who have sex with other
men in addition to having sex with women; see Campbell 1990; Hutchinson 1993), and most injecting drug users (IDUs) and most hemophiliacs

are men. Male bisexuality has become a major factor in transmitting HIV to women throughout the Americas. This is especially so in places where exclusive homosexuality in men seems to be less common than it is in North America, such as parts of South and Central America. A survey conducted in Mexico of more than five thousand men who have sex with men found that 56 percent of the sample living in Mexico City also had sex with women. The frequency of bisexuality was 51 percent in other large cities and 67 percent in medium-size and small cities. Moreover, 35 percent of the men surveyed had stable heterosexual relationships. In Lima, Peru, a survey of 354 men, conducted in public places frequented by men who have sex with men, found a 30 percent frequency of bisexuality. Bisexual men used condoms more often with male partners than with female ones, and had lower levels of perceived AIDS risk than the heterosexual men surveyed (De Bruyn 1992).

I should note here that, while many studies conducted with homosexual men in the United States suggest that the risk of infection is positively related to the number of sexual partners (Walker 1991, 108; see Bolton 1992 for a counter-argument), it is probably not the "one-night stands" that transfer the infection to women. After reviewing the literature, Margaret Nichols concluded that multiple partnering may increase a woman's risk for other sexually transmitted diseases and thereby render her more vulnerable to the transfer of HIV into her bloodstream during or just after sex with her primary partner; nonetheless, Nichols found no relationship between the number of sexual partners and seroconversion (1990). She suggests that more women are infected by steady male partners than by one-night stands or casual liaisons (see also Reiss 1991, as cited in Bolton 1992). This is because, programmed by safer sex campaigns that denounce and vilify multiple partnering ("promiscuity") and advise us to "know" our partners, most couples assume that monogamy confers protection from HIV and so do not maintain safer sex standards (Bolton 1992).

In addition to the biological and sociodemographic factors linked to being female, the tenor of gender relations and the structure of gender-linked power differentials affect women's risk for infection with HIV. For instance, trying to reduce one's risk of exposure by asking a male sex partner about his sexual history or serostatus may afford a woman less protection than such a strategy affords a man. In a study of the use of lying in the negotiation of safer sex, men were significantly more likely than women to admit having lied (35% versus 10%) (Cochran 1989).

Gender-based power structures, which in mainstream U.S. culture are intimately linked with ideals for heterosexual relations, affect male-female communication. They affect what transpires in the sexual arena, and so affect women's chances for HIV infection.[1] Because of these power structures and relationship ideals, women often find themselves in positions in which not all sexual options are equal and not all risk taking is voluntary.

My use of the phrase "risk taking" needs qualification. As Martha Ward observes, "Risk taking implies autonomy in the world" (1993a, 427) — an autonomy that many women lack. This is especially true for the impoverished, and Ward suggests that "given the power differentials in contemporary society it may be sensible to think of HIV in poor women as vertical transmission instead of horizontal transmission" (427; technically, vertical transmission is the transmission of HIV from parent to child; horizontal transmission occurs between sex partners assumed to be consenting equals).[2]

Poor Minority Women

On the public level, more attention has been paid to women as infectors of men and children than as infectees themselves, and, although things are changing, more AIDS-related projects are aimed at helping white men and children than dark-skinned women (Bezemer 1992). Even in predominately minority neighborhoods, most resources go to male IDUs or gay men of color (Cochran and Mays 1991). But women of color, most of whom are in their childbearing years, comprise the fastest growing group of HIV-infected people. Three-quarters (74.6%) of U.S. women with AIDS are members of minority groups.

The majority of U.S. women with HIV infections or AIDS are poor, Black, and living in urban areas (CDC 1993c). Blacks, about one-eighth of the U.S. population, account for over half of all U.S. women with AIDS. Black women are about sixteen times more likely than white women to be diagnosed with AIDS (CDC National AIDS Clearinghouse 1995). By the end of the 1980s, the death rate among Black women between the ages of fifteen and forty-four was nine times that of white women in the same age range (Chu et al. 1990 as cited in Hutchinson 1993).

In light of these statistics, it is tempting to single out Blacks as a "risk group" — a bounded group that, by virtue of some essential trait, is at a high risk for AIDS. The notion of the risk group is an artifact of early responses to the AIDS pandemic, which included the epidemiological identification of four specific subsets of people in whom AIDS was most commonly diagnosed: homosexuals, heroin users, hemophiliacs, and Haitians. Specific subsets of the world's population are indeed at a higher risk for contracting AIDS. However, this has more to do with social history than with ethnic, national, sexual, or other aspects of one's identity. So while these aspects of identity may serve as risk markers they are not, in themselves, risk factors (JAMA 1993).

The risk-group model encourages flat, essentialist explanations and appeals to the notion of monolithic cultural beliefs (Glick Schiller 1992; Kane and Mason 1992). In my work, I consider diversity among Black women; the research described here seeks to distinguish those who practice safer sex from those who do not. It also seeks to examine Black women's beliefs and behaviors against the broader U.S. cultural context rather than as isolated, culturally determined phenomena, because, despite intergroup differences, high-risk behavior in the United States cuts across ethnic, class, sexual identity, and other so-called boundaries.

The psychosocial forces related to unsafe sexual practice (described in detail in Chapter 7) probably exist universally, albeit to greater or lesser degrees in different sociocultural contexts. But the conditions of life in U.S. inner cities make unsafe sex among those who live there particularly likely to lead to HIV infection. Economic oppression (and its effects on gender relations), substandard health care, the frequency of IV drug use, high rates of untreated venereal infection, and other typical inner-city and poverty-related conditions exacerbate the effects of unsafe sexual practices on the rate of HIV transmission among Black and other inner-city women (Mays and Cochran 1990; Ward 1993a; Worth 1989). For this reason, the concerns of poor urban women must receive high priority on the AIDS prevention research agenda.

The Sexual Arena

Black Female Sexuality

Most of the ethnographic data presented in the chapters below were collected through the self-reports of Black women and fit well with the existing literature on Black sexuality. As will be made clear, certain findings give the already-published information new significance by revealing previously hidden and unexplored patterns, while other findings contradict old assumptions about the link between money and love.

My review of the existing academic literature on the sex lives of poor urban Blacks will be brief, partly because little in-depth documentation exists. We have a fair amount of information concerning contraception among Black women and girls, but most of this is only quantitative; moreover, contraception is just one area of sexuality. The research I describe later helps answer the call spurred by the AIDS pandemic for more data on Black sexuality (see Institute of Medicine 1988, 193; Muir 1991, 77; Turner et al. 1989, 109).

Some of the other works generated in response to this call consider rates of various sexual practices among Black women. Despite the liberal amount of public attention Blacks reportedly give to sex (Fullilove et al.

1990), research demonstrates that many Black women are conservative during actual sexual encounters. Repertoires are limited (Wilson 1987; Worth 1990) and rates of certain kinds of high-risk sexual practices are lower among Black than among white women (Lewis and Watters 1989; Weinberg and Williams 1988).

In a study involving a representative sample of 8,500 U.S. women of childbearing age (15–44), Seidman et al. (1992) found multiple sexual partnering to be rarest among never-married Black women.[3] In a background paper for a National Institutes of Mental Health and of Drug Abuse (NIMH and NIDA) workshop, Wyatt et al. (1988, as cited in Turner et al. 1989, 113) reported that Black women are half as likely as whites to recount ever having had anal sex (21% for Blacks; 43% for whites). The majority of urban minority women who participated in a study by Kline et al. "voiced strong objections to anal sex" (1992, 454), and both Fullilove et al. (1990) and Wyatt and Dunn (1991) found that Black women were more likely than white women to prefer vaginal intercourse. Worth (1990) speculates that this preference may have to do with a greater procreative orientation. It also may be linked with sex-related guilt, which Wyatt and Dunn (1991) found to be significantly higher among Black than white women. Further, Wyatt and Dunn found that Blacks, especially of lower income, held less permissive attitudes in relation to premarital sex than whites (regarding contradictory findings among Black men, see Fullilove et al. 1990; Weinberg and Williams 1988). However, Fullilove et al. (1990) note that, among lower-income Blacks, women's sexual aggression or assertiveness toward men, rather than premarital sex per se, is frowned upon.

In a study of sexual dysfunction carried out with lower-income inner-city women in Cleveland just before I arrived there, House et al. (1990) found that the mean frequency with which Black participants said that they desired sex (1.83 times weekly) was less than that for whites (2.06 times weekly).[4] No other significant variations between Black and white women were found, but, as these women were drawn from the same pool as participants in my study, some of the other findings bear repeating. For instance, the mean reported frequency for actual intercourse (2.71 times weekly) was similar to the mean frequencies reported elsewhere for wealthier samples of Black and white women, as well as for other samples of lower-income Black women.

As House et al. note, "In most respects the data suggest that the sexual behavior of [the] sample is quite similar to that of middle-income women" (1990, 172). Like many middle-income women, 10 percent of the participants in the study had never experienced an orgasm. Of the women who reported having orgasms with their partners, the orgasms occurred an average of 52 percent of the time that they had intercourse.

As for the intercourse frequency figures, the orgasm statistics for the lower-class Cleveland women were similar to those reported in other studies and for women of other income levels. However, the figures for masturbation were not: they showed that lower-income women masturbate far less than women with higher economic standing.

So, while some of the differences between Black and white female sexuality are culturally determined, other so-called differences are not cultural differences at all but instead are socioeconomic artifacts (cf. De La Cancela 1989; Kline et al. 1992; Ward 1993a).[5] Increasing Black acceptance of cunnilingus and other shifts in Black women's sexual patterns (Wilson 1986; Wyatt et al. 1988) supports the argument that the sexual habits of Black and white women are beginning to converge. Wyatt et al. explain that Black women's changing sexual tastes "tend to be a function of [their] assimilation . . . into the American mainstream" (1988, 329).

Materialist Models and Gender Tensions

Most of the existing literature on sex among Blacks focuses on the economic and structural reasons for a perceived cultural emphasis on the instrumental dimension of sex, and sex among urban Blacks often seems to have little to do with love and emotion. Conjugal ideals are frequently presented as being categorically different from mainstream, middle-class (i.e., white) norms (e.g., Mays and Cochran 1988; Worth 1989; Fullilove et al. 1990), but, as I argue later, this may not be the case (cf. Anderson 1990; Cochran 1989; Oliver 1989; Stack 1974).

While the basic heterosexual conjugal model held by Blacks may actually be quite similar to that held by whites, the intergender sexuality-related differences among Blacks are high (e.g., Anderson 1990; Fullilove et al. 1990; Mays and Cochran 1990; Worth 1990).[6] Fullilove et al. argue that Black men are oriented more toward the erotic, Black women more toward the romantic (1990). But perhaps the most glaring and widely reported difference is that partnered men are expected to have active extraconjugal sex lives while women are not. Weinberg and Williams (1988) report that 76 percent of Black men have had at least some extramarital sexual experience; 30 percent of Black men have had more than five extramarital sex partners, not including prostitutes.[7]

Like most statistics regarding extraconjugal sex, these numbers refer only to married men. However, many Black couples are unmarried. Nearly 40 percent of unmarried Black men have multiple partners (Bower 1991).[8] Regarding Black urban men in particular, Geringer et al. (1993) found that nearly half of their study participants had had sex with casual partners in the six months preceding the study. In the four weeks preceding, each man had had an average of two sexual partners.[9]

It is important to note that heterosexually coupled men can cheat bisexually (Muir 1991, 91; Turner et al. 1989, 152). Covert bisexuality is thought to be more common among Blacks than among European Americans because of the ways Black identity is constructed. Many Black men who have sex with men give their primary allegiance to the Black community rather than to the gay community, and as members of the Black community they are expected to engage in heterosexual relations (Dalton 1989; Mays and Cochran 1990; Wilson 1986). Among bisexuals with AIDS, Black men are "dramatically overrepresented," accounting for 28 percent of all cases (Mays 1989, 266); Black homosexual and bisexual men engage in higher rates of active and passive anal sex than their white counterparts (Bell 1978, as cited in Mays and Cochran 1987).

The high level of non-monogamous heterosexual intercourse culturally recommended for and often achieved by Black men is generally traced to their lack of economic opportunity and their related dependence on favorable peer evaluations (Anderson 1990; Liebow 1967). William Oliver explains the "complex of values and norms that characterize the way many lower-class Black males define manhood" — a complex that includes "the tough guy and the player-of-women images" — as a "dysfunctional cultural adaptation to white racism" and a "compensatory adaptation" (1989, 260–61). Following Hannerz, he calls this "compulsive masculinity" (Hannerz 1969, as cited in Oliver), and argues that lower-class Black men's adherence to norms emphasizing sexual conquest contributes to intergender conflict, which itself often results in male-on-female violence. Male-on-female violence, says Oliver, is one of the reasons that Black married couples get divorced twice as often as whites.[10]

An orientation toward sexual conquest and a sex ratio of 92 unmarried men aged eighteen through thirty-nine for every 100 unmarried women in the same age range (Johnson 1993, 52) encourages men to take many mates. Sometimes brought up hearing that "half a man's better than none," women frequently ignore infidelity and share partners with other women. This practice limits the social, emotional, and (sometimes) financial resources available to each woman, sometimes leading them to take many mates, too.

Women's Sexual and Reproductive Strategies

Although economically disadvantaged women are often forced by circumstance to engage in what Marie Muir calls "survival sex" (1991, 153), female non-monogamy can be used as a strategy of empowerment.

Dooley Worth's findings indicate that a large proportion of poor urban women establish extraconjugal relationships because their primary partners do not satisfy them emotionally or sexually (1989). But multiple partnering among women has generally been analyzed primarily as a strategy to expand resource bases (e.g., Freilich 1968; Handwerker 1993; Stack 1974; see also Worth 1989). Even having children, which involves unprotected sex, can be understood this way, given the lack of alternatives or career opportunities for many women.

Men are often eager to sire offspring because babies provide proof of their "manly" heterosexual activity (Anderson 1990; Liebow 1967). For women, having a baby can be an attempt to improve one's status: each child born holds the promise of achieving great things and reflecting well on the mother (Mays and Cochran 1990) as well as of being a source of joy and unconditional love. Also, women can have children to please and bind men — to establish structural links with them. Children enable women to establish other sorts of structural links as well: having a child is a prerequisite for membership in many female support networks (Ward 1990). Knowing this, and also knowing that the supply of marriageable or employed men is small due to the frequently cited high rates of imprisonment, death by homicide, and unemployment among Black men, some women choose to build families and network connections without the perceived burden of a husband or boyfriend (Wilson 1987).

Sex and the Risk of Infection

Unprotected sex, necessary in many cases for male support (whether social, emotional, or financial) and always needed for conception, entails HIV risk. It also entails risk of infection with other sexually transmitted diseases. In 1980, two-thirds of all reported U.S. cases of syphilis and gonorrhea were among Blacks, with Blacks suffering 45 times as much syphilis and 34 times as much gonorrhea as whites (Johnson 1993, 98, 151). A Black woman who has unprotected sex with a Black man from an area where sexually transmitted diseases (STDs) are endemic takes a big risk that she will contract one — and STDs are often cofactors in (or enablers of) HIV infection because they create sores where HIV can enter and exit.

A woman's HIV risk level depends on many factors in addition to her STD history. These include geography, drug use, income, and various factors affecting risk perception, evaluation, and acceptance. As has been widely noted, HIV is just one of many dangers faced daily by impoverished urban minority women. When coupled with inner-city conditions, Black constructions of sexuality support many women's conclusion that the only way not to do worse "is to take risks to do better" (Wildavsky

1988, 226). As Fischoff et al. argue, the "choice of an option depends upon all of its features, not just its risk" (1981, 124). The benefits of heterosexual interaction and of possible motherhood outweigh the risk of disease when *not* risking this could lead to more immediate consequences such as verbal or physical abuse, the loss of a partner, or childlessness (cf. Pinkerton and Abramson 1992; Shervington 1993), consequences that involve not only tangible hardships but also lowered status and damaged self-esteem.

While "self efficacy," which refers to one's perceived capability of executing a behavior or making a behavioral change (Bandura 1977), has been associated positively with AIDS-risk reduction (Turner et al. 1989, 279), dysphoria or hopelessness among inner-city women has been associated with low levels of insistence on safer sex (Orr et al. 1994; Tunstall et al. 1991). Women's perceptions about their options and about male-female status disparities may negatively affect their constructions of self efficacy, thus decreasing their sexual decision making and communication power. This in turn diminishes women's ability to introduce innovations such as condom use into the sexual arena. The power structure inherent in heterosexist conjugal relations does the same (Copelon 1990; Muir 1991, 153; Schneider 1988). Yet, as Kline et al. (1992) point out, and as I demonstrate, despite cultural ideals regarding female subordination, "minority women often retain substantial power vis à vis their male partners with respect to sexual decision making. Factors relating to perceptions of risk are frequently more salient barriers to the practice of safer sex in this population" (1992, 447). In any case, few of what AIDS educators would call sex-related risk-reduction steps are consistently taken by impoverished urban Black women.

Women with AIDS

Woman's Illness Experience, Man's World

As the AIDS pandemic gained a foothold in the United States, it was perceived as a problem affecting only men. The CDC's list of diseases indicative of AIDS and their criteria for a positive diagnosis reflected this misperception. Because women's bodies are different from men's, AIDS in women often presents itself in what was, according to CDC criteria, a nonstandard fashion. Many women were misdiagnosed; others went from doctor to doctor in search of an answer or a label for their suffering that nobody could give (as did many PWAs prior to the biomedical recognition of the syndrome). Even when it became apparent that HIV was not a sexist germ and that the possibility of a female patient's being infected by it should be examined (regarding HIV antibody testing, see Chapter 8), diagnoses for women were usually delayed, as they often still are, particularly among poor people of color. And delayed diagnoses mean delayed therapeutic action, which can hasten death.

After January 1, 1993, when the CDC amended the official definition of AIDS to include opportunistic infections likely to strike women (such as invasive cervical cancer), the number of women diagnosed with AIDS increased dramatically: 204 percent more women were diagnosed with AIDS in the first three months of 1993 than in the same time period in 1992 (CDC 1993a, 3). Gaining status as a PWA has important effects on the range of financial and other assistance available to the ill individual. So classified or not, lower-income women infected with HIV frequently have pressing medical and social welfare needs. The following discussion of how these are handled draws heavily on findings from Martha Ward's work in New Orleans (1993b).

As Ward observes in regard to Black urban women, "The diagnosis of HIV only adds another bureaucracy and another layer of complications to an already burdened life" (1993b, 59). This is partly because "the programs for women do not have the vitality or originality of those for gays; they are only puny grafts on an already overtaxed health care system" (61). Moreover, in the experiences of urban women, the health care system is not user-friendly (cf. Lazarus 1990). This is especially true when users have HIV/AIDS, which, as Peggy McGarrahan explains, "Both because of its nature and because of the patients affected [people of color, IDUs, homosexuals], has made visible the fragmentation and disarray of the health care system" (1994, 29).

HIV is not generally an infected inner-city woman's worst problem; as Ward found, there are often other sick people in the family and children to feed and rent to be paid. Like most mainstream women, inner-city women with HIV often feel that they must take care of others before they take care of themselves. And indeed, often they must; as Nina Glick Schiller writes, "It is the unpaid, undocumented health services provided by female kin that allow the health care industry to carry on" (1993, 489).

Women frequently find it easier to bring a sick child to the doctor than to go in for their own appointments (and while some clinics have recently tried to batch or consolidate appointments for the convenience of their clients, adults and children often must go to different clinics, on different days). Clinicians are often more sympathetic toward pediatric AIDS cases than they are toward equally sick women. Ward writes of "cases where many service providers, professionals, and volunteers attend the funeral of a baby dead from AIDS; not one of them is present at the mother's funeral" (1993b, 60). Clinicians, like lay people, often blame the women for infecting their babies and themselves through what is seen as careless, stupid behavior.

Even for inner-city women who do have the energy and time both to take care of themselves and to deal with accusing attitudes, quality health care is often beyond reach. As Janis Hutchinson points out, "Access to health care in the US is usually dependent on ability to pay for it" (1993, 10–11). In addition to health care not covered by what little insurance she has (if any), an ill inner-city woman must find a way to pay for transportation to appointments, child care, and so forth. Prescribed drugs are usually prohibitively expensive. Furthermore, many of these have not been tested on women, as their susceptibility to HIV infection and AIDS was ignored until recently.

Besides problems linked to class and gender, HIV-positive women of color seeking health care must contend with racism, which is pervasive in the health-care system. As Hutchinson (1993) notes, racism exhibits itself in cursory physical examinations, deficient bed assignments, delayed admissions, and assumptions of noncompliance; further, it often overlaps with class-based discrimination against the poor, and influences the adoption, implementation, and administration of health policies that limit certain aspects of the lives of lower-income people. In a recent study of AIDS outpatients, Moore et al. (1994) found significant disparities between the frequencies with which certain drugs were prescribed to urban Blacks and whites, regardless of income or insurance status. Blacks seem to have received less follow-up care as well. Because some clinicians think Blacks are noncompliant, they prescribe certain therapies less often for Blacks than they do for whites.

Therapeutic issues notwithstanding, confidentiality is a major concern for most infected women. For caregivers, clients' desires to control knowledge of their infections pose logistical headaches (for example, remembering which relative or family friend is not to be informed of the real health problem) and ethical ones, especially when clients are minors or when their children have AIDS. "The strictures of confidentiality often apply to an afflicted baby's grandmother even when she is the primary care giver," says Ward. "In some cases, the grandmother is told only that the baby has a rare blood disease" (1993b, 60). Their concerns about confidentiality lead most HIV-positive women to shy away from using the services of supportive community organizations, which they view with suspicion and see as intrusive and possible spreaders of gossip.

Mays and Cochran point out that impoverished Black HIV-positive women may emphasize secrecy more than other seropositive people do because "the impact of rejection for Blacks may be more severe, given existing cultural norms emphasizing the kinship network as the provider of both tangible and emotional social support" (1987, 227). Infected mothers may feel that their kin will be more likely to care for their children after they die if the cause of death is kept secret. Seropositive women often remain secretive to guard their own lives as well as their children's; some fear that, if told, their male partners may leave them, abuse them emotionally or physically, or even murder them. At least two women have been shot for their seropositivity and "many others" have been injured (*Baltimore Sun* 1993; regarding serostatus self-disclosure, see also Chapters 4 and 9).

AIDS and Reproduction

While seropositive mothers worry about what will happen to their children after they are dead, HIV-positive women are frequently faced with decisions about whether to bear children in the first place. Many women learn that they are infected only after being tested in the course of prenatal care (testing and women's attitudes toward it are discussed in depth in Chapter 8). If there is time, pressure is often put on them to undergo abortion; however, many poor women do not seek prenatal care until their pregnancies are well underway (Lindsay et al. 1990; regarding barriers to prenatal care, see Lazarus 1990).

 All babies carry maternal antibodies, and so all babies born to HIV-infected women carry their mothers' antibodies for HIV. All these babies will look at first as if they are infected. But in nearly three out of four cases the HIV antibodies disappear after about fifteen months (as do other maternal antibodies). So an infected woman's chances of giving birth to a healthy child are actually relatively high. Treating the mother-to-be with the anti-AIDS drug azidothymidine (AZT) may increase these chances further (CDC 1994b),[11] although its expense puts it out of reach for many inner-city women. But even the odds of three out of four babies being healthy are not bad in light of the other obstacles inner-city women face daily. These odds and the joy that a child can bring in the future lead many HIV-positive pregnant women to carry their babies to term (testimony regarding childbearing from HIV-positive people is provided in Chapter 9; see also Campbell 1990; Catania et al. 1990; Carovano 1991; Levine and Dubler 1990).

Other factors also encourage childbearing among HIV-positive women. Current legal restrictions, social and cultural pressures, financial problems, and some clinicians' fears of exposing themselves to HIV make getting an abortion very difficult for seropositive inner-city women who would choose to do so (cf. Levine and Dubler 1990). Further, the woman faces not only the excrutiating loss of a future child, but also other social losses. Partners, friends, and family members aware of the pregnancy may demand an explanation for her decision, and revealing her seropositivity may result in abandonment.

Abortion-related social losses can go beyond immediate relations;

abortion is, to some, a tool for genocide. Levine and Dubler write that, "Efforts to stem the spread of HIV through the control of reproduction may be seen as attempts to destroy the African-American and Latino communities" (1990, 334). They also point out that

HIV infection, as one of a range of conditions that can be passed from mother to fetus, should not be particularly singled out for moral censure and coercive policies. Other, less stigmatized conditions are equally or even more likely to be transmitted, to result in suffering or death for the child, and to be costly to the family and society. (1990, 322)

Further, as HIV-positive women may be motivated by love for a soon-coming baby to try to change their sexual habits (Tunstall et al. 1991), asking them to forgo motherhood involves forfeiting what Mays and Cochran have called "the 'teachable moment.' " That is, with abortion a woman gives up a potential child that might have been a "serendipitous motivator" for health-seeking action (1988, 953; see also Levine and Dubler 1990).

AIDS in women is, as Ward says, a "different disease" from AIDS in men (1993a). Not only is female biology different, leading the disease to take a different course, but women's lives and the challenges that they face are different too. Poverty and racism compound the significance of those differences in the inner city. The next chapter examines the factors that, as with pregnancy, may contribute to AIDS risk reduction behavior among women. It also discusses the factors that act as obstructions against it.

Notes

1. Class, ethnic or race, and age disparities that can exist between partners also affect sexual decisions and behaviors.

2. In light of Ward's point about poor urban women's relative powerlessness, we might also question the appropriateness of referring to mother-to-child transmission in poor urban settings as vertical. For calling it such implies that the mother controls the infection of the child, when, in light of Ward's point about poor urban women's lack of autonomy, it cannot be so simple.

3. Multiple sexual partnering was most common among divorced or separated Black women (Seidman et al. 1992). However, Seidman's figures must be interpreted in light of the fact that many inner-city Black women never marry.

4. Because the sample was small and no statistically significant differences existed for other variables, interpretations of these findings must be made with caution.

5. Weinberg and Williams (1988) argue that consistent and significant differences persist between Black and white men regardless of their socioeconomic standings. The differences they show between Black and white women are fewer,

but according to Weinberg and Williams they are nevertheless associated with ethnicity, not with socioeconomic status.

6. The intergender sexuality-related differences among Blacks seem to be greater than those among whites (Weinberg and Williams 1988).

7. These estimates were based on data collected by the Kinsey Institute.

8. So do 40 percent of white men (Bower 1991).

9. 99 percent of the men were sexually active at the time of the study, 90 percent with primary partners.

10. According to Oliver, Black men murder four times as many women as white men do. The latter generally live in different political and economic circumstances than the former; accordingly, intergender relations have a different cultural shape (1989, p. 267).

11. The possible long-term effects of AZT on infants are not known (although the effects on adults are known often to outweigh the benefits). It may be that maternal-infant AZT therapy significantly raises infants' risks for cancer and other health problems in the long term.

Chapter 3
AIDS Education and the Perception of Risk

The research for this book grew out of the concern that Cleveland's Maternity and Infant Health Care Program (M&I) clinic clients were not heeding the M&I safer sex message. There was nothing unique about the relative failure of the M&I AIDS education mission, which focused on the dissemination of factual information. Most studies conclude that no significant relation exists between safer sex and the degree of AIDS or HIV knowledge people have (e.g., Farmer and Kim 1991; Geringer et al. 1993; Johnson 1993; Linden et al. 1990; Mays and Cochran 1988; Prohaska et al. 1990); behavioral changes made by homosexual men (Turner et al. 1989, 136) living in areas with firmly established gay social and political structures are the exception (see Winkelstein et al. 1987). But even among this group patterns of relapse have been documented (Miller et al. 1990, 109; Stall et al. 1990). Factual information is necessary, but it is certainly not sufficient to drive and sustain behavioral change. This chapter asks why not, and investigates the key role risk perception plays in motivating (or obstructing) health-protecting behavior such as condom use.

The Failure of Education

AIDS "Facts," AIDS "Myths"

Findings from the 1992 National Health Interview Survey (Schoenborn et al. 1994) indicate that 96 percent of U.S. adults know that HIV can be transmitted through sexual intercourse and 94 percent know that it can pass from pregnant women to their babies perinatally; 96 percent know that it is "very likely"[1] that an individual will contract HIV if sharing needles with an infected person. Among Black Americans the respective percentages are lower, but only by one to two percentage points (regarding AIDS knowledge levels of Blacks in particular, see also Flaskerud and

Rush 1989; Hardy and Biddlecom 1991; Harrison et al. 1991; Jemmott and Jemmott 1991; Johnson 1993).

People do have the facts, but they do very little with them. One of the most common problems in prevention education is that the facts about HIV and AIDS are disembodied — they are not presented in relation to the health ideas clients already hold. As a result, people often have done little more than memorize the "AIDS facts" they are taught. Once memorized, this information is easily regurgitated in response to questions such as those posed on surveys meant to measure AIDS knowledge levels.

As Irving Zola points out in relation to health surveys in general,

> We may be comforted by the scientific terminology if not the accuracy of [the respondent's] answers. Yet if we follow this questioning with the probe: "Why did you get X now?" or "Of all the people in your community, family etc. who were exposed to X, why did you get . . . ?" then the rational scientific veneer is pierced and the concern with personal and moral responsibility emerges quite strikingly. Indeed, the issue "why me?" becomes of great concern and is generally expressed in quite moral terms of what they did wrong. (1972; ellipses in the original)

The masked beliefs can concern more than just morality (as discussed later). Often, old health beliefs have not been set aside or replaced but instead simply have been augmented. Accordingly, while AIDS knowledge levels among Blacks, for example, are generally high, many still fear doorknobs and public toilets because "you never know" (Flaskerud and Rush 1989, 212; see also Hardy and Biddlecom 1991; Schoenborn et al. 1994). The educatees memorize the scientific explanations of the AIDS educators, but traditional means of contagion still operate in many people's minds as science and tradition co-exist.

In a study of AIDS knowledge and risk behavior among women from a range of ethnic groups, Harrison et al. (1991) found that, while the majority of participants possessed reasonably accurate AIDS information, many still believed that casual contact can spread AIDS (cf. Becker and Joseph 1988; Kimmel and Keefer 1991). For example, when asked whether one could contract AIDS through shaking hands or kissing cheeks, or through insect bites, many women answered incorrectly. Eleven percent of the Hispanics, 28 percent of the whites, 32 percent of the U.S. Blacks, and 36 percent of the Haitians thought that kissing and shaking hands could spread HIV infection. Twenty-three percent of the whites, 32 percent of the Hispanics, 34 percent of the U.S. Blacks, and 42 percent of the Haitians thought that insects such as mosquitoes could transmit HIV as they went from person to person.

Harrison et al. (1991) attributed the latter belief among Haitians to traditional beliefs concerning illnesses caused by spirits (the researchers did not discuss the possible causes of the existence of the insect-bite belief among the other groups of women, nor did they talk about hand-shaking or cheek-kissing beliefs). Throughout African Caribbean society, people consider the body permeable and believe that spirits cause illness by various means, including by penetrating the body through open pores or other orifices. Many U.S. Blacks share similar beliefs (Snow 1974). In fact, cross-culturally, most health traditions include some form of per-meability model. Permeability models make sense: pores do open and close, and bodies do incorporate matter (as through eating or receptive condomless sex) and they expel it, as through sweating, vomiting, lactat-ing, menstruating, and urinating (see Sobo 1993b). Even modern bio-medical discourse refers to a permeability model, for example, in refer-ence to airborne germs, which we breathe in through our mouths, or other germs such as HIV, which we take in through other bodily open-ings. Traditional and modern biomedical health beliefs can easily coexist and in fact often sustain one another.[2]

That people memorize new "facts" but still retain old ones does not mean that most AIDS educatees lack the ability to think critically. As Leventhal et al. note in their discussion of the ways that people generate common-sense representations or models of illness, people "attempt to understand and to regulate their medical treatment. It is incorrect to conceptualize the patient as a passive object who needs to be pushed to action" (1977, 15). So, being active participants in their own lives, AIDS educatees make what use they can of the materials and concepts provided by AIDS educators. For example, educatees may be admon-ished to "refrain from the exchange of bodily fluids" without being told what that phrase means or which fluids in particular to avoid (Becker and Joseph 1988; Turner et al. 1989, 263). They must use existing explanatory models of illness (e.g., the permeability model) if they are to make sense of this "AIDS fact."

Comprehensibility

Sometimes approaches to AIDS education are incomprehensible to the common client. Although education methods are being overhauled, many brochures used in AIDS education campaigns are written at the college level, while many people seeking AIDS information from public clinics have not yet completed high school (the average participant in my study in Cleveland had left school in the eleventh grade). Furthermore, brochures providing self-tests for clients to rate their own risk levels often undermine the safer-sex message they intend to promote. Neil Weinstein explains, "Because few people will score high on all risk factors, such brochures may decrease the sense of risk for most individuals," leaving them with a false sense of security, and without the desire to implement condom use and other precautions (1989, 156).

As Victor De La Cancela (1989) notes in reference to the effectiveness of AIDS intervention campaigns, the mode of communication chosen must be prestigious and trustworthy. Accordingly, another problem with using brochures in Black neighborhoods is that many Blacks may be more comfortable with radio and television than with printed matter (Mays 1989). Mays reports that Black women spend more time than whites watching television or listening to the radio; Blacks have much less hostility toward television and perceive its contents as being much more credible; they are also more likely to use television as their primary information source. In this light, De La Cancella's recommendation of the use of Black-associated music, videos, and television soap operas to get the safer-sex message across makes good sense. For this to work, local dance hall DJs and Black-oriented radio and television stations (especially those that broadcast to predominately Black neighborhoods) must be involved in the anti-AIDS campaign.

Cynicism

AIDS-education messages must be formulated in a manner sensitive to the fact that, in addition to some confusion about modes of transmission, many people have understandable doubts about standard prophylactic recommendations and about the infallibility of biomedical experts and public health officials. Findings from the 1990 National Health Interview Survey (Hardy and Biddlecom 1991) indicate that only slightly more than one in four Blacks (27%) view condoms as "very effective" for the prevention of AIDS, while 44 percent see them as "somewhat effective." Moreover, Black women feel even less sure than Black men that condoms protect well against HIV transmission: while about one in three Black men (35%) feel sure, just over one in five Black women (22%) do.

Participants in my condom use research (described in detail in Chapters 5–8) voiced their own suspicions about the prophylactic value of condoms, backing these up with references to current scientific disagreements, media reports about very real problems with condoms, and propaganda promoted by groups like the Nation of Islam (cf. Thomas and Quinn 1991). They also supported their skepticism with stories about personal experiences of condom failure, which certainly does happen (Steiner et al. 1993; Thompson et al. 1993).

Moreover, participants pointed out that unprotected sex is just one of many ways that a person may catch AIDS; for example, HIV might be transmitted in an emergency blood transfusion, or by a vindictive individual (one who malevolently conceals his serostatus or pokes a hole in a condom to infect a woman without her knowledge; see Chapter 4). Most participants had second-hand stories about situations in which such accidental or purposeful transmission occurred. This kind of extrapunitive or attributional thinking—in which others can infect us with HIV no matter what we do—releases us from culpability or responsibility for our health, but it lends no support to safer-sex practices because it means that infection can come at any time and in any way—not just through unprotected sex (or indiscriminate needle-sharing). Accordingly, it makes little sense to "spoil" sex by introducing condoms. That condoms are not foolproof only adds to the apparent futility of trying to use them.

Some Black cynicism regarding condoms and the safer-sex message has to do with a historically low level of trust in the health care system. This distrust, to which I shall later return, hails back to slavery days when, as Dooley Worth writes, sick slaves were subjected to "many official or 'white' medical practices that were actually damaging to their health" (1990, 125–26). Many blacks fear discussing AIDS in public health settings because they believe white staff members will use the information to hurt them or blame them for health problems.

Facing not just racism but a whole hierarchy of daily risks (cf. Mays and Cochran 1988; Worth 1989), many poor urban Black women find the effort to have safer sex nonsensical or excessive. This is especially true for those who see AIDS as largely unavoidable. On many days, tasks like putting food on the table, finding employment or getting transportation to work, keeping one's children safe from harm, keeping the apartment warm, or even simply finding time to go to the Laundromat before it gets dark and dangerous outside take precedence over worrying about a disease that could take years to surface.

Self-Sabotaging Logic

Ralph Bolton (1992) notes that, although change is coming, most AIDS education programs currently take a two-pronged approach. On the one hand, they recommend condom use in the context of multiple partnering, casual sex, or an unfaithful lover. On the other hand, they advise against multiple partnering, implying or stating outright that monogamy is the surest protection against HIV (although this is probably not the case). The first recommendation is problematic because people may not trust condoms or even the idea of them, for reasons just discussed. Condom promotion also begs the question of safer sex: the emphasis on condoms (as opposed to other safer-sex methods) suggests that penetrative-receptive sex should be practiced, when to evade HIV transmission it is actually best avoided. Further, as Bolton notes, this "approach is negative and critical rather than empowering," and emphasizes danger rather than pleasure (61).

The second element of the typical approach implies that monogamy is an alternative to or substitute for safer sex, and suggests that who you have sex with (e.g., your husband or the postal carrier) is more important than what you do (e.g., anal sex or mutual masturbation) and how you do it (e.g., with or without a condom) (cf. Kline and Strickler 1993). Notwithstanding that the emphasis on monogamy fails to take real sexual patterns into account, clients put off by the sex-negative messages surrounding condom use can instead focus on (accept) the recommendation to maintain monogamous relations which, according to the logic of the intervention message, excuse them from safer sex.

Clients can easily shift their focus in this way because mainstream U.S. culture generally idealizes monogamy. Furthermore, as Bolton argues, the vague advice to "know your partner" creates "the perception that it [is] safe to have sex with people one [knows] because they couldn't possibly be infected" (1992, 39). Bolton suggests on the basis of his research that it is to a large extent this kind of advice that causes most women who get AIDS to be infected by long-term rather than casual partners (see also Nichols 1990). Bolton argues that, because of "the net loss of life that has occurred as an unintended consequence of the dual-pronged strategy" (56), all anti-promiscuity messages should be excluded from AIDS education curricula.

Applicability

Standard AIDS education programs have an idealistic focus on monogamy, as if they seek "to reconstruct a hegemonic mythical paradise in which sex [occurs] only within marriage" (Bolton 1992, 59), failing to take into account alternative or divergent cultural constructions of sexuality and relationships. While many groups share the mainstream U.S. model of heterosexual conjugal relations (monogamous, etc.), certain aspects of this model as presented in AIDS education interventions draw too heavily on white and Western middle-class values to be applicable in the inner city. For example, as Mays and Cochran (1990) point out, advising women to talk with their partners during sex presupposes a companionate model of conjugality that may not, in reality, be applicable to many poor urban Black couples (although it may be desired). Promoting safer sex with ads that characterize sex as play and present it in a vacation-like framework may alienate Blacks who do not view sex in that fashion or who may not have the time and the privacy to enjoy sex in that way; and it may alienate religious Blacks. Also, assuming that having children is unimportant may alienate not just religious women but those for whom having a child will be one of the most creative, life-affirming things they can do.

When assumptions behind safer-sex models have little to do with the reality experienced by the clients targeted for "education," some of the information dispersed will be dismissed or reinterpreted in terms of the clients' own beliefs about the situations and outcomes in question.[3] Awareness of clients' constructions enables educators to communicate better, safeguards against misinterpretations, and facilitates clients' adherence to health recommendations. Kleinman et al. discuss this issue in an explication of the clinician-patient interactions that constitute "clinical realities" (1978, 254). When one party says one thing, the other party may hear another, or may misunderstand or even reject — overtly or covertly — what was stated, because the parties bring different assumptions to their meeting.

Education programs must maintain sensitivity to gender issues, cultural rules regarding sexual expression and conjugal or intimate relationships, and cultural models of health. They must present the facts about HIV transmission and AIDS more clearly and more simply so that people understand completely what should be done to increase their safety. And they must teach people how to maintain behavioral change (De La Cancela 1989). For example, taking the client's household or network as the primary unit of treatment rather than treating her as an isolated individual can improve adherence to recommendations.

The level of support offered by a client's social circle influences his or her health behaviors (Medalie et al. 1981; Schmidt 1978; see also Turner et al. 1989, 291–93). So does the level of commitment that the client feels toward that circle. Altruism has been identified as a factor in the reduction of AIDS-related risk behavior among injecting drug users (IDUs) and homosexual men (Turner et al. 1989, 279), and women may seek HIV safety for their children more quickly than they do for themselves (Tunstall et al. 1991; see also Ward 1993b).

The individualistic focus of white culture sometimes makes little sense to Blacks, for whom social responsibilities often come first (Mays and Cochran 1990). Accordingly, AIDS educators might also increase client response by involving grass-roots community organizations and respected community members, which builds credibility (De La Cancela 1989).

Condom Accessibility

Even with the above education program modifications, and even if fail-safe condoms that fit all sizes comfortably become available, condom use will not suddenly increase unless condom distribution patterns are altered. Currently, in many clinics, people must walk up to the receptionist's desk and, in front of that receptionist and everybody else, collect a week or two's supply. This can be quite intimidating and demoralizing. A unique study that allowed drug abuse clinic clients to collect condoms from a private clinic restroom as well as from a public clinic waiting room found that 381 percent more condoms were taken from the restroom (Amass et al. 1993). Clearly, private access to condoms is an important issue.

Risk (Mis)Perception

Reasoned Action and the Role of Emotion

I have just traced a logical argument or outline regarding the shortcomings of current AIDS education strategies, using the common Western paradigm of rationalism. Because of the sovereignty of logic in Western thought, the models most frequently used in predicting health related behaviors and designing interventions assume that reason motivates people's actions. Examples of models emphasizing rational client cognition include the Health Beliefs Model (Janz and Becker 1984) and the Theory of Reasoned Action (Ajzen and Fishbein 1980), both of which have been explored in relation to AIDS (Fishbein and Middlestadt 1989; Jemmott and Jemmott 1991; Kirscht and Joseph 1989). The axiom of rational action supports the hypothesis that people will want to use condoms if they can logically conclude that the benefits of condom use outweigh the costs.

Many who forgo condoms have not even gotten as far as considering the condom's utility.[4] They reject safer-sex practices out of hand, thinking that they are simply not at risk for HIV infection. Perceived susceptibility (perception of risk) is a key variable in the aforementioned Health Beliefs Model; it also figures, although not so prominently, in the Theory of Reasoned Action and in the more recently formulated AIDS Risk Reduction Model (Catania et al. 1990). These models acknowledge that a person's perception of his or her risk for the health threat in question plays a significant role in his or her response to that risk.

Including perceived susceptibility in health-seeking models like these assumes that individuals who correctly perceive that they are at risk for a health problem will want to take steps to avoid it.[5] In the case of AIDS, however, research has confirmed that understanding the risks that might lead to AIDS does not automatically engender safer-sex behavior, because, no matter how well informed they are, people tend to underestimate their own risk for AIDS (Carovano 1991; Harrison et al. 1991; Hansen et al. 1990; regarding low perceived susceptibility to STDs in general, see Geringer et al. 1993).

AIDS and the major modes of transmission often associated with it —
anal sex and intravenous drug use — are highly stigmatized by mainstream U.S. culture. For many, just thinking about AIDS and these actions mobilizes negative affect: it stirs up bad feelings, such as guilt,
shame, or even hostility and disgust. Negative affect limits our ability to
correctly perceive risk. Admittedly, even without emotional interference,
most people are incapable of correctly calculating probabilities in their
heads because of the complex mathematics involved and the myriad
factors that must be considered (insertor or insertee past history of STDs;
partner's STD history; area of residence; partner's area of residence;
partner's current drug-use habits; partner's past drug-use habits; etc.).
Accurate perceptions of AIDS risk are beyond our cognitive capabilities.
But emotion exacerbates the situation by making certain kinds of cognitive errors, such as optimistic bias (which I explain below), much more
probable.

Some rational action models of health seeking, such as the AIDS Risk
Reduction Model and the Health Beliefs Model, explicitly acknowledge
the mediating effects of emotion on risk perception, but none examine
the mechanism behind it. None explain exactly how emotion comes to
encourage or motivate cognitive errors. Research focused specifically on
risk perception suggests that the emotions and meanings associated with
a given risk affect perceived susceptibility. They influence the way people
do or do not personalize, internalize and apply to themselves the information they receive about that risk (Weinstein 1989; see also Hansen et
al. 1990). That is, emotional reactions affect how we will apply what we
learn to ourselves.

"Optimistic Bias" and AIDS-Risk Denial

Generally, people who think "AIDS can't happen to me" believe that,
although HIV is virulent, nothing they are doing or have done puts them
at risk for infection. Objectively, this may not be so, and various factors
like where one lives and one's partner's sexual and drug-related habits
affect one's objective chances of contracting HIV. In any case, and no
matter what the objective level of risk, in the context of mainstream U.S.
culture, believing or indicating that one is at risk for AIDS involves admitting one's shameful or immoral failure to live up to standards for prudent
sexual (or drug-related) comportment. Because disclosing such a failure
can have dire effects on self-esteem, identity, and status, many people
engage in what Neil Weinstein (1989) has called "unrealistic optimism"
in regard to their risk for AIDS. That is, many maintain optimistically
biased states of AIDS-risk denial. (Regarding AIDS-risk denial's link to
"robust" mental health, see Joseph et al. 1989.)

I use the expression "AIDS-risk denial" to refer to the outcome of cognitive error, as cognitive mistakes (whether emotionally motivated or simply failures in calculation) lead people to underestimate their risks and so to deny or disown them.[6] The expression also applies to mentally defensive AIDS denial, that is, the process by which we remove from our conscious thoughts threatening ideas about being at risk for HIV infection. The mental discomforts thereby avoided can include cognitive dissonance (when a certain piece of information clashes painfully with or calls to question what is already known) and emotional disharmony (when a certain piece of information provokes intense anxiety or fear regarding one's reputation or one's relationship).

The latter kind of denial — defensive denial — does not happen every time cognitive or emotional threats occur; often, depending on the context and nature of the threat, people can work through and even resolve anxieties or cognitive dissonances without having to repress them. Further, defensive denial is not an all-or-nothing process; its degree of intensity can vary over time and situationally. But when the disharmonic threats are too large or too disturbing — for example, if they threaten to undermine our culturally constructed view of the world and of our place in it — we tend to deny them. We do this in order to maintain our mental health and preserve our self-esteem and social position.

Self-Esteem and Status

Relevant cultural knowledge and information about role expectations is essential for predicting when and how specific kinds of denial will occur, and for developing strategies to combat this denial. In the case of AIDS, denial of risk enables one to escape frightening thoughts of one's susceptibility, social marginality, and impending physical and even social death. Further, denying AIDS risk allows a person to preserve self-esteem and status, just as admitting risk by using condoms can lower self-esteem (see Worth 1989). Denying one's risk for AIDS involves covertly or overtly denying that one engages in the stigmatized, culturally unacceptable practices likely to lead to HIV infection.

The implicit assumption here is that a person desires to preserve his or her social standing; that is, he or she values or "buys into" the culture's stance on sexuality and conjugal relations (of course, some people do not, and my argument does not apply to them). We are also assuming that the person has the emotional strength required to use the optimistic bias in defense of his or her social standing. For instance, depressed individuals are less likely to claim low vulnerability to given outcomes because, being depressed, they have lost the motivation to preserve their self-esteem (Weinstein 1984).[7]

By denying risk, people not only preserve but also can raise their status and self-esteem: denying one's own risk implicitly—and sometimes explicitly—involves asserting that others are at a higher risk. Indeed, people often report that their peers' risk levels for negative outcomes like AIDS are higher than their own, which they see as comparatively low. They tend to assume that their own self-protective actions are more extensive or effective than others', perhaps simply because they know and understand their own self-protective actions better than those of others. Further, people tend to compare themselves to stereotypes who take few or no self-protective actions (high-risk individuals) rather than to their actual peers (Weinstein 1989, 1982; cf. Kinsey 1994). They tend to compare themselves to a construct of the " 'average person' . . . who is, almost by definition, less advantaged, less intelligent, and generally worse off than oneself. Consequently, it is perhaps not surprising that subjects judge themselves as more immune to negative events than the average person is" (Perloff and Fetzer 1986, 503).[8]

Even people aware of their own high risk for AIDS tend to engage in biased comparisons that lead them to conclude that their peers' behavior is more risky than their own (Weinstein 1989). Importantly, this kind of slanted interpretation is not simply an artifact of an express concern over others' opinions. Optimistically assessing one's risk as lower than the risks of one's peers occurs whether or not one expects to be compared to others by an outside judge—the expectations of the inner judging self suffice (Weinstein 1984).

Katherine Kinsey (1994) studied the HIV and AIDS related knowledge, attitudes, and beliefs of about one hundred urban women who received AIDS counseling and education, most of whom were members of minority groups. Kinsey observed participants' use of what she called "distancing maneuvers" to maintain denial. For example, one participant said, " 'I know four brothers (all drug abusers) who have AIDS but I don't do what they do and besides they live in a different neighborhood' " (83; parentheses in original). Participants also used their own negative HIV test results to support optimistically biased, self-esteem-affirming contentions that they were not at risk for contracting the virus.

The women's reasoning patterns did not draw on the HIV and AIDS related facts they had learned, which they knew but did not personalize or internalize. Instead, their reasoning centered on their personal experiences, or what Scott Rushforth calls "primary epistemic evidence" (1994). Rushforth contrasts the "primary knowledge" built on such evidence with the disarticulated and impersonal "secondary knowledge" provided by expert systems such as biomedicine. He explains that in certain contexts a high reliance on primary knowledge and an active distrust of expert systems serves as a form of resistance to intrusive or dominating forces associated with those same expert systems.

Optimism, Preventability, and Shame

Risk-related optimistic bias appears to be a universal phenomenon, unaffected by age,[9] gender, education, or occupation. Further, optimism occurs in relation to minor problems as well as to life-threatening risks; it seems unrelated to the perceived seriousness of the risk (Weinstein 1987).[10] Both in general and in relation to AIDS, optimistic bias does not correspond with a person's actual risk level; the mechanism at work among high-risk individuals also is at work among low-risk people (regarding general risk, see Weinstein 1984; regarding AIDS risks, see Hansen et al. 1990; Weinstein 1989; see also Prohaska et al. 1990; Shtarkshall and Awerbuch 1992). Optimism does, however, have a strong correlation to a risk's perceived preventability (Weinstein 1984, 1987, 1989).

Most people see AIDS as preventable. Because optimism in risk perception corresponds positively with the degree of preventability (and so of potential personal culpability) ascribed to the condition being considered, AIDS is a prime candidate for optimistic bias. Weinstein has noted that "People tend to be unrealistic about their vulnerability to hazards perceived to be controllable" (1984, 439). As he writes, "The more preventable the hazard, the greater the threat to self-esteem" (1989, 157), and the greater the threat to self-esteem, the more useful optimistic bias can be.

We often recall our risk-decreasing actions while forgetting our risk-increasing actions. Two factors underlie this forgetfulness. First, people tend to keep their thoughts about their behavior and their thoughts about their vulnerability "in quite separate mental compartments" (455). When trying to evaluate risk, they must recall and integrate the information stored in these "mental compartments." In doing so, says Weinstein, "Risk-decreasing actions might come to mind particularly easily because they are often conducted for the explicit purpose of reducing risk. Risk-increasing actions, in contrast, are seldom carried out to intentionally increase risk" (444), and so they are less likely to be accessed. For example, people can easily recall having been selective about past sexual partners—a strategy that, if correctly carried out, should negate the risk-increasing potential of condomless sex (but often does not, as shown below). The negative HIV test results recalled by the participants in Kinsey's (1994) study also exemplify the sort of information easily within cognitive reach.

Second, especially in the case of AIDS as it is such a stigmatized and fatal condition, participation in risk-increasing actions might be pushed out of awareness to maintain a sense of mental ease. Fear of death, for example, can be dissipated in this way. More important perhaps, so can fear of disgrace: optimistic bias corresponds positively with the degree to which a person expects to feel greatly ashamed if she or he develops AIDS (Prohaska et al. 1990). The more stigmatized a condition is, and the more people think that the condition can be avoided by taking precautions, the more likely people are to underestimate their risk for that condition. This is due to the impact that the fear of disgracing oneself (and perhaps one's family) and the other bad feelings generated by thinking about the threat (e.g., of AIDS) have on the severity of the cognitive error called the optimistic bias.

Findings on HIV test outcomes and self-reported risk factors demonstrate the problematic nature of AIDS-risk perception. Landesman et al. interviewed and HIV-tested 602 poor urban non-white new mothers in New York (1987, as cited in Nichols 1990). Two-thirds of the women who tested positive did not suspect that they were at risk. Similar findings were reported by researchers in Atlanta who tested 3,472 inner-city minority women during pregnancy (Lindsay et al. 1989). Each woman filled out a brief questionnaire to assess her risk for HIV infection. Had the researchers only tested women with self-reported risk factors, as per official recommendations, "more than 70% of [the] seropositive women would not have been identified, because they did not self-acknowledge risk factors" (293).[11]

Partner Selection as a Self-Protective Strategy

The sizable optimistic bias that is generated in a large part by the stigma attached to AIDS and its perceived preventability is also encouraged by current AIDS education techniques. As noted, AIDS educators generally stress the importance of monogamy and of choosing one's partner carefully. They suggest implicitly, then, that condoms are not necessary with honest fidelity because monogamy confers sufficient protection from the spread of HIV infection. Like most U.S. women, most Black women agree with this assumption because, on a certain level, it makes sense. Backed by the standard discourse on selectivity and monogamy, many women seem to use information-seeking strategies to reduce their chances of selecting an HIV-positive partner in the first place. The "safe partner strategy" (as defined, for example, by Metts and Fitzpatrick 1992), consists of selecting a partner from among friends, and assuming that "unsafe" people are somehow distinguishable. "Most individuals," say Metts and Fitzpatrick, feel that they are indeed "heeding the warning to know their partner as a way to practice safer sex" (4; see also Maticka-Tyndale 1992; Pivnick 1993). As a participant in Kinsey's study said, "If I pick a good man, one I think is clean, then I know I'll be OK" (1994, 83).

As I shall show in Chapter 7, once the selection of a mate is made, many monogamy-minded women optimistically attribute adulterous instincts only to other women's men. They do this partly to avoid cognitive dissonance (disharmony between particular thoughts or ideas) and emotional pain. Armed with the knowledge provided by AIDS educators, these women can logically conclude that they themselves not at risk for HIV infection.

Community Level Risk (Mis)Perception

Risk and Group Pride

Risk is perceived not only in relation to oneself, but also in relation to one's membership in a given community. The idea of acting to reduce HIV transmission has been, for many Blacks, what Ernest Quimby calls a "culturally circumscribed existentialist absurdity" (1992, 160), partly because, as Quimby notes, "Poor health is a structural feature of Black existence" (161). In other words, most Blacks are poor and this, along with the racism that it is tied to, severely limits the health care options open to Blacks while greatly expanding their health challenges (see Lazarus 1990; Ward 1993a).

 However, the unfeasibility of community AIDS-risk reduction efforts also stems from many Blacks' belief that as a group they are not at risk for AIDS. This opinion (which is changing as Black AIDS tolls rise) is not confined to disempowered women, with their culturally and structurally promoted dependence on maintaining the sexual patterns described in Chapter 2. I have argued that the popular (albeit misguided) associations between AIDS and immoral sexual depravity, deviance, and foolish risk-taking can diminish people's willingness to recognize that their own behavior puts them at risk for infection, as doing so would signal personal inadequacy. The negative connotations of AIDS also diminish the willingness of whole communities of people to see that their own members might be infected, as admitting this in the context of current AIDS-related attitudes would signal a community's inferiority and inadequacy. Like individuals, whole groups of people can deny that they are at risk for HIV infection if it benefits them to do so.

Harlon Dalton (1989) and Ernest Quimby (1992) show that community-level AIDS-risk denial among Blacks is part of a self-protective strategy adopted in the face of racist finger-pointing and blame-laying (regarding this strategy and non-U.S. Blacks, see Farmer 1992). As Quimby explains, "potential embarrassment" (179) serves as a major deterrent to "owning" AIDS and so to dealing with AIDS risk; HIV and AIDS are reminders of "cultural disenfranchisement," "political feebleness," and

the fragility of social mobility (178). For many Blacks, risk denial is essential for group pride and support of equal rights claims.

Conspiratorial Thought

Group dignity can also be supported with conspiracy theories. These
generally hold that AIDS is part of a secret germ warfare plan. In his book
examining the tendency in the United States to blame Haiti for AIDS and
investigating the Haitian response to that charge — a response that involves counter-claims concerning conspiratorial plots (e.g., as devised
and executed by the U.S. CIA or FDA) — Paul Farmer explains AIDS
conspiracy theories as rhetorical defenses employed by people with little
power (1992, 231–32, 247).

In the United States, some claim that AIDS was created by the "White
Establishment" and launched against Blacks as part of an extermination
plan (cf. Turner 1993). Those who believe this argue that, because they
are targeted to die, Black "AIDS victims" cannot be blamed for their
sickness. Some also say that HIV infection is unavoidable, because the
White Establishment will find a way around self-protective acts, perhaps
by putting HIV in prelubricated condoms or using HIV test needles to
inject the virus directly into the blood of the target-group members.[12]
This theory casts Black "AIDS victims" as innocent and helpless. Further,
since population growth is a way of insuring that a people will not be
silenced or die out, some Blacks who see AIDS as part of a deliberate
attempt at genocide will advocate condomless sex because it permits
conception. Unsafe sex becomes an act of resistance to oppression.

The Genocidal Plot

In September 1993, as I outlined my plans for this book, an individual posted a note on the electronic bulletin board of the sci.med.aids
network[13] inquiring about the theory that HIV was "man-made." The
sci.med.aids network is one of a number of AIDS networks, consisting of
lay people and AIDS specialists. Most sci.med.aids dialogue concerns
scientific understandings of AIDS or HIV and the progression of AIDS,
but now and then a simple query as to whether or not you can "catch
AIDS" through kissing does appear.

The question about the human invention of AIDS was posted by an
amicable, articulate man named Mr. Green.[14] He asked for information
about the White Establishment's conspiratorial role in creating HIV
for the specific purpose of "offsetting the growth rate of Black people
around the world." He explained that, according to an unspecified article in the (Black militant religious group) Nation of Islam's periodical

The Final Call, a (white) scientist in California altered a cattle virus to invent a virus very similar to HIV. The article apparently also said that some people think that HIV was spread in Africa in the 1970s through polio vaccination programs. Mr. Green was fairly well convinced by what he read, and wanted to know more. Perhaps he assumed that sci.med.aids readers were familiar with the conspirators' activities.

Most readers ignored Mr. Green's plea. Some of the few who did post responses were unnecessarily impolite; others more civilly referred Mr. Green to specific papers reviewing popular theories regarding the origins of AIDS. I wrote directly to Mr. Green asking for more information. One of the more interesting things he told me was that Louis Farrakhan of the Nation of Islam wrote (again, in an unspecified article in *The Final Call*) that a doctor in Africa had discovered a cure for AIDS. Farrakhan allegedly claimed that the cure for AIDS—a disease supposedly aimed at annihilating Black society—involved a substance from the pituitary glands of adolescent Black males.

This type of assertion also is reported by Patricia Turner, who identifies it with a *genre* of popular Black discourse called the "castrated boy legend" (1993, 163). This label notwithstanding, the statement attributed to Farrakhan effectively claimed that Black males full of potent, youthful, life-affirming, and life-creating sexual desire and substance would save the world through the biomedical assertion of their virility. According to Turner's work, such a claim is not unique: "The dominant population's need for physical components of the minority population is common in folk discourse" (149).

The Final Call is just one of many sources promoting or reporting the idea that AIDS is part of a plot against Blacks. Some of these sources are esoteric, arcane pamphlets procured through the mail or at specialty bookstores and passed from hand to hand; others are easily accessible to huge groups of people. A series of stories in the *Los Angeles Sentinel,* the largest Black newspaper on the West Coast, promoted the idea that Blacks have been infected with HIV intentionally (see DeParle 1990; Guinan 1993[15]). An article entitled "AIDS: Is It Genocide?" (Bates 1990) was published in *Essence,* a magazine tailored for Blacks. *Newsweek* carried a story exposing "An American History of 'Plans' for Blacks" (Cary 1992), and the popular television show *Tony Brown's Journal,* often shown on Public Broadcasting System (PBS) stations, aired a series of debates over the genocide theory (Guinan 1993). Such media coverage fuels the transmission of conspiracy rumors by exposing wide audiences to them and providing them with an aura of authenticity.

Conspiracy theories held by people of African heritage about AIDS and other STDs have been discussed in the academic literature (e.g., Dalton 1989; Jones 1992; Quimby 1992; Thomas and Quinn 1991; Turner

1993), editorialized in the *New York Times* (e.g., 1992; see also DeParle 1990) and *Newsweek*, and documented for Africa (Walker 1991), Haiti (Farmer 1992), and Jamaica (Sobo 1993b), as well as for the United States. Anecdotal accounts scattered throughout social-scientific writings on AIDS, discussed in the above-mentioned critical and theoretical writings, and encountered in my own research (e.g., the focus-group data mentioned above in relation to condom use cynicism) support the contention that a significant number of people have heard of the "AIDS Conspiracy."[16] But a 1993 search of the academic literature turned up only one short report (Guinan 1993). Interestingly, the findings described suggest that genocidal thinking is not limited to militant or Afrocentric Blacks (see also DeParle 1990).

In the report, Guinan (1993) presents data from research conducted by the Southern Christian Leadership Conference (SCLC), founded by Dr. Martin Luther King. The SCLC is one of several community organizations receiving funds from the CDC for AIDS education and outreach. On receiving funding, the SCLC surveyed Black church leaders regarding their attitudes toward and knowledge of AIDS. About two in three respondents (65%) thought it possible that AIDS is a form of genocide; more than one in three (35%) felt sure of it. "Now, if this selected, educated population thinks that AIDS is a form of genocide," asks Guinan, "then what does the rest of the community think?" (193). Had the study involved a random sample of Blacks, Guinan contends, a much higher percentage of believers in the genocidal theory would have been found.[17]

A 1994 search of the academic literature turned up another study of conspiratorial thought, the results of which supported Guinan's suspicion. Gregory Herek and John Capitanio (1994) examined Black cynicism regarding AIDS in the context of a larger project dealing with AIDS stigma. Using a national telephone survey, they found that two in five Blacks (43%) believed information regarding AIDS is being held back from the public; one in four (27.5%) distrust experts regarding casual contact; and one in five (20%) agree that the government is using AIDS to kill off members of minority groups.[18]

Other Kinds of Plots

Ideas about genocidal plots against Blacks represent one specific variant of the "AIDS Conspiracy." Some versions concern the withholding of information or the dissemination of misinformation. Others posit homosexuals as the population targeted for annihilation; still others blame the conspirators' ineptness for the pandemic. Many stories share several elements. In some accounts, genocidal ones included, the unheeded findings of so-called "AIDS experts" (most of whom mainstream scientists regard with disdain) are cited extensively to legitimate the claims. In other accounts, the links to "Science" or to existing theories are implicit.

According to some rumors I discovered through the Internet, AIDS comes from dairy products. The idea that we are being poisoned through the food that we eat may be common: participants in the focus groups held during the first phase of my own study also told tales of an infected food supply. Some believed that "the AIDS virus" is in the meat that we eat; after all, agribusinesses often pump up animals' flesh with chemicals (e.g., the hormone DES). It is not impossible that HIV may have somehow gotten mixed in with animal feed. Many participants said that fish from Lake Erie is especially likely to be contaminated; after all, the lake is polluted with "man-made" chemicals which easily could include HIV. Eaten or absorbed by fish, HIV could be passed on to the humans that in turn consume the fish. Participants did not agree whether this contamination was accidental or the result of a conniving plot; many women argued that government officials had warned against eating fish caught in the lake, a fact that indicated they did not intend to harm the people.

Regarding cattle, one Internet rumor was that Canadian scientists had traced a particular strain of HIV back to a particular dairy. Another rumor held that the U.S. government has long known that AIDS comes from tainted dairy products but has hushed it up for years. This rumor may be a subtle twist on the aforementioned cattle virus rumor that Mr. Green described, itself possibly linked to a school of thought promoted by certain men working, ostensibly, from within the scientific community (although not from a respected corner of it).

The ideas of Robert Strecker and Jakob Segal have provided much grist for conspiracy rumor mills.[19] Segal argues that HIV was formed from the sheep virus visna and human T-cell leukemia virus (HTLV-I) by U.S. Army biological research laboratories in the late 1970s. It escaped accidentally after being tested on prisoners. Strecker argues that HIV was formed from visna and bovine leukemia virus (BLV) by the U.S. in the 1970s after between thirty and forty years of work.[20] The U.S. government supposedly tested the virus on specific groups of Africans, introducing the virus through smallpox vaccinations produced from viral lesions of experimentally infected cattle (Bates 1990).[21] They then deliberately introduced it into the U.S. homosexual community through the hepatitis B vaccination program.[22]

The viruses implicated in Strecker's and Segal's theories are all retroviruses. Retroviruses have three subfamilies: oncoviruses, lentiviruses, and spumaviruses. HTLV and BLV are oncoviruses. There are two branches of lentiviruses: nonprimate lentiviruses, of which visna is one, and primate lentiviruses, which include HIV-1, HIV-2, found in humans, and simian immunodeficiency virus (SIV), found in certain kinds of monkeys and baboons. So BLV, HTLV, and visna are quite different from HIV. HIV and visna, the alleged key in the "germ warfare" sequences described by Strecker and Segal, do have similarities as both are lentiviruses, but HIV and SIV have much more in common (C. Jonsson, personal communication; see also Cullen 1991).

Further evidence against Strecker's and Segal's ideas includes the fact that, although they each set the date for the so-called invention of HIV in the 1970s, HIV has been found in preserved blood samples from the 1950s. Moreover, biotechnology was not sufficiently advanced in the 1970s to produce anything like HIV, and it is debatable that it would be possible even now, especially since the details of HIV and many of its operations on the human system are still poorly understood. And while the military do deal in "germ warfare" studies, they have historically been interested in "germs" to which people have no natural immunity, not "germs" that destroy the immune system.

Finally, data on the incidence of AIDS in sexually active homosexual men undermine Strecker's claim that HIV was introduced into the homosexual population via hepatitis B vaccinations. According to a study carried out in the early 1980s, the incidence of AIDS in unvaccinated men was actually slightly higher than in vaccinated men (rate differences did not reach statistical significance) (McDonald et al. 1983). In a second, slightly later study, about 6½ percent of a blood sample set from the beginning of the vaccination program was found to be already HIV-positive, indicating that HIV could not have been introduced via the vaccinations (Stevens et al. 1986).

According to the CDC Clearinghouse (1993; see also Weiss, 1994), the spread of the rumor that a U.S. military science "germ warfare" experiment led to the development of HIV was underwritten by the Soviet KGB, which promoted its spread as part of a *dezinformatsiya* campaign that lasted from 1983 until 1988. Soviet disinformation practice generally involves expanding on and promoting legends that already exist in seed form. Some of the details added to the "germ warfare" rumor by the Soviets included the name of the supposed development site (usually said to be Fort Meade in Maryland) and the claim that HIV was invented during attempts to create a plague that would kill only non-whites. This rumor was circulated in twenty-five different languages and in more than eighty countries, including European and developing ("third world") nations. The campaign might have been launched in retaliation for the Reagan administration's claim that a biological weapon controlled by the Soviets had produced yellow rain (rain associated with the yellow traces found on vegetation, which have since been attributed to natural causes).

The Legacy of Mistrust

While one theory holds that the purposeful infection of Africans was a prelude to the purposeful infection of male homosexuals in the United States, another theory, promoted by City College of New York (CCNY) Black Studies professor James Small, among others, holds that homosexual white men were the real guinea pigs. As *Essence* reporter Karen Bates wrote, they "were merely a test batch, the practice run for the real target: us [Blacks]" (1990, 78). Leonard Jeffries, who heads CCNY's Black Studies Department, also has gone on record stating that AIDS is part of a plan for exterminating Blacks.

Researchers tend to link Black fears about AIDS and genocide directly to Black knowledge of the historic and exploitive Tuskegee Syphilis Study (see Jones 1992; Thomas and Quinn 1991; Turner 1993).[23] The study, which began in the pre-penicillin year of 1932, involved documenting the natural course of untreated syphilis in about 400 poor Black men. The men were manipulated into participating in the study with false promises of free medical treatment and financial incentives.[24] Media exposure of the study in 1972 led to its termination and, ultimately, to the passage of the National Research Act in 1974. The Act mandated that proposals for all federally-funded research involving human subjects be submitted to and reviewed by institutional review boards, which may reject any proposals deemed unethical or scientifically misguided.

Here, I must point out that a number of common beliefs about the Tuskegee Study are erroneous. On learning about the study, people often assume that the participants were intentionally infected with syphilis (my own students often assumed this and, as Guinan noted in 1993; so did Yale law professor Harlon Dalton, who perpetuates this distortion in his 1989 article on AIDS and Blacks, p. 220). While their assumptions may be incorrect, the feelings and knowledge that lead people who hear about the Tuskegee study to draw biased conclusions often stem from actual life experiences. And, as James Jones points out, the study's existence validates perceptions of racism and maltreatment in such a way that people who learn about it often cling to it as "a symbol of their mistreatment by the medical establishment, a metaphor for deceit, conspiracy, malpractice, and neglect, if not outright racial genocide" (1992, 38).

Personal experience of racism and the legacy of negative encounters Blacks have had with the public health system fuel the misgivings that many Blacks have about health care workers' motives and intents (Guinan 1993; Jones 1992; Thomas and Quinn 1991; Worth 1990; regarding racism coupled with sexism and class discrimination, see Corea 1992; Lazarus 1990). In regard to AIDS, inner-city Blacks — perhaps especially inner-city Black women who, because of their childbearing and caretaking roles, have more experience with the health care system than men — recognize the questionable quality of the health care available to them. They know from personal experience the health care delivery system challenges faced by the disenfranchised (Ward 1993a; cf. Corea 1992; Lazarus 1990).

Intragroup Differences

While most Blacks have experienced the kind of maltreatment and discriminatory deception that feed conspiratorial thought, intragroup differences (such as those related to age and gender) affect the ways group members experience oppression and victimization. Consequently, the degrees to which subsets of Blacks subscribe to conspiracy theories should vary, as should the content of these theories. This was the case among those who participated in the focus groups held during the first phase of my research, to be described in full in Chapter 5. I have mentioned these focus group discussions in relation to the often cynical reception that education efforts can meet, and to the meat and fish rumors. Members of the three focus groups also talked about the origins of AIDS.

Many women reported having heard of laboratory accidents, contaminated water, or withheld information. Four men were visiting when origins were discussed, two each in two groups and none in the third. While the men spoke openly of AIDS as part of a racist plot to eliminate Blacks, the women generally did not. They may have ignored race in order to maintain an identification with the researchers, most of whom were not Black, while gender differences between the men and the researchers, all of whom were women, may have left the men free to attend to color. But issues related to race were broached by women at other points in the discussions, suggesting that women may simply be less likely than men to advance racist conspiracy theories.

Women do experience racism and are well aware of the possibility of genocide. But Black men and women interacting with white society encounter different kinds of barriers to social mobility, self-esteem, and status. It may be harder for Black men to fulfill cultural expectations to provide for their families than it is for Black women to fulfill cultural expectations to be mothers. This difference may affect the rhetorical needs of each gender, and so may influence the content of the conspiracy theories subscribed to by each.[25] In addition to gender, age also may play a mediating role.

Rhetorical defenses and self-esteem enhancing strategies are played out both on the individual, intragroup level and on the community, intergroup level. While conspiracy theorizing protects group esteem, individual risk denial protects self-esteem. In the latter case, by accepting the notion of individual responsibility and then rejecting or denying one's individual risk for HIV infection, as we do in optimistically biased risk assessments, a person can enhance or preserve her own self-esteem and raise her intragroup status.

As fits with the principles of segmentary opposition (Evans-Pritchard 1968), which posit an ongoing social dynamic of context-linked group fission and fusion, people whose group pride is threatened by AIDS-related accusations join together in exhibiting community-level risk denial or resorting to conspiracy rhetoric to deny individual ability to avoid AIDS. However, in the context of intragroup relations people highlight individual responsibility for preventing HIV infection and exhibit optimistically-biased personal AIDS-risk denial. Self-esteem and status are thereby bolstered and sustained, and frightening thoughts about the shame and social death that would accompany AIDS, not to mention the physical pain, need not be confronted. The immediate mental health advantages of maintaining denial and persisting in high-risk behavior have been documented for gay men by Joseph et al. (1989), who note that "robust" psychological well-being seems incompatible with accurate risk perceptions. I believe the same holds true for inner-city women. The last half of this book will examine denial's individually self-protective function in relation to idealized cultural constructions of gender and of heterosexual relationships. But first, I shall briefly discuss seropositivity self-disclosure.

Many individuals fear that sex partners may be lying to them when they promise that they are not infected with HIV. The next chapter explores this fear, discussing the problems and issues confronting seropositive people as they consider how to tell their intimate partners about the illness — and whether they should tell them at all.

* * *

Much of the material in this chapter was adapted from "Inner-City Women and AIDS: The Psycho-Social Benefits of Unsafe Sex," *Culture, Medicine, and Psychiatry* 17(4) (1993):455–485 and "Finance, Romance, Social Support, and Condom Use Among Impoverished Inner-City Women," *Human Organization* 54 (2) (1995):115–128.

Notes

1. The needle transmission question was not a yes-no question, as the perinatal transmission and sexual transmission questions were, but used a Likert-type scale.

2. Before beginning the study described in later chapters, I thought that health-linked understandings about sex would be tied to the avoidance of condoms. I suspected that participants would hold explanatory models of AIDS transmission that would prove significant in regard to their sexual behavior (cf. Flaskerud and Rush 1989). Like the women in the sample surveyed by Harrison et al. (1991), many participants in this study did overestimate the number of ways that HIV can be transmitted. People also suggested the fact that AIDS results from a virus, as does a cold or flu, implies that AIDS is treatable. The "virus" label lessened the perceived severity of the syndrome for some. But no distinct or highly developed explanatory models emerged. The participants' health ideas about AIDS were nebulous and limited to simple contagion models implicating casual contact (e.g., handshakes, shared drinking vessels, etc.), much like the models that seem to be held by most U.S. citizens. Ideas linking sex and physical health also proved limited. Only one of the 18 first-phase interviewees agreed that sex is necessary for good health. Nearly one in four simply disagreed, and one in six actively countered the assertion, citing negative physical effects ("too much sex ages you"; "if it had to do with health, no diseases would be out there") and noting that celibate people are no worse off physically than highly sexed ones. Less than half thought that men need more sex than women; a thirty-six-year-old mother of six commented, "Men *think* there is a difference [in drive and] culture allows this." She also observed, "The only pride [Black men] have is sex," which she explained as being due to racist conditions. The only interviewee who linked sex to physical health said that it benefits the heart; significantly, the heart is traditionally associated with love. While this particular participant did not make this connection explicit, three in four women referred specifically to the emotional functions of sex. They frequently described sex as a relaxing act that "clears the mind." As it "helps you sleep" and relieves tension that can manifest itself physically, sex does have bodily effects; but these were linked to emotional rather than physical health enhancement.

3. I had hypothesized that knowing a person with AIDS (PWA) would be associated with risk-reduction among participants, as it was for a group of homosexual and bisexual men studied in the epidemic's early years (McKusick et al. 1984). Participants themselves proposed that people would adopt safer-sex practices if they knew PWAs. The intuitively logical nature of this assumption has led to few tests of it. In both the first-phase interview and the focus group survey, participants were asked whether they knew any PWAs. Nearly one in four focus group women did, consistent with Gerbert et al. (1991) in which one in four African Americans (24.2%) knew PWAs. But twice as many interviewed as surveyed focus group women reported knowing PWAs. Self-selection might explain this; focus group members knowing PWAs may have been more motivated to be interviewed. But knowing a PWA was not related to frequent condom use among participants. Other studies have also found no relationship between knowing PWAs and condom use or personal vulnerability worries (Pivnick 1993; Zimet 1992). Without generalizing, it is worth noting that the focus group women who reported knowing PWAs were actually more likely to engage in unsafe sex than those who did not know PWAs: three quarters who knew PWAs used condoms "never" or "rarely," while only half of those who did not know PWAs did so. Perhaps knowing PWAs encourages hopelessness, which in turn leads to a lack of interest in risk reduction (Orr et al. 1994; Tunstall et al. 1991). Alternatively, and in keeping with the main findings of this study, increased risk taking may be a form of denial aimed at maintaining one's self-image of invulnerability and wisdom. (Or maybe those

who know PWAs belong to social networks that, on the whole, engage in high-risk sexual practices more often than members of other social networks; indeed, people who know PWAs seem to be more tolerant of homosexuality [Gerbert et al. 1991].) AIDS-risk denial also spurred focus group members' intense expressed interest in discovering how known PWAs contracted the disease; participants looked for blatant carelessness on the part of each PWA against which to compare favorably their own (underplayed) risk taking. This helped them to cling to their optimistically-biased belief that "It can't happen to me."

4. One reviewer indicated with a red pen mark that I had forgotten an "f": the word "futility" made more sense to her here than the word "utility" did. However, since utility may be valanced as negative or positive, while futility carries only negative connotations, I thought it best to stick with the original word choice.

5. Recognition of personal risk can have psychological costs (Joseph et al. 1989); it can lead to despair and has even been associated with increased risk taking (Kirscht and Joseph 1989). For this and other reasons, perceived risk is only a peripheral part of the Theory of Reasoned Action (Fishbein and Middlestadt 1989). Despair and fatalism seem to be linked with low levels of perceived "self-efficacy," which has been identified as an important factor enabling intentional behavioral change; it is now part of most health behavior models (regarding the concept, see Bandura 1989). However, when susceptibility is not perceived even those with the highest measurable levels of self-efficacy will take no risk-reduction steps.

6. Regarding the computation of AIDS-related underestimation factors, see Shtarkshall and Awerbuch 1992.

7. In the case of AIDS, depression may be the result rather than the cause of accurately perceiving one's risk for infection (Joseph et al. 1989).

8. In distancing themselves from the comparison group, people may protectively resist acknowledging their friends' and family members' vulnerability (Perloff and Fetzer 1986).

9. While others have reported that age does correlate positively with increased AIDS risk denial (e.g., Hansen et al. 1990), the recent literature on adolescent risk taking suggests that the age-eighteen dividing line our society sees as the significant delimiter of youths from adults is based on criteria that are inapplicable to the urban poor. One assumption we use to differentiate youths from grownups is that youths take more risks, believing themselves to be immortal or invulnerable. But, as Susan Millstein (1993) argues, there is no empirical support for the claim that teens are more likely than adults to think in this fashion. Millstein compared data from a number of sources and found that youths were no more likely than adults to have optimistically biased perceptions of risk. The same was true for other kinds of perceptual and inferential risk assessment biases. Further, in a study of age-specific mortality rates, Charles Irwin determined that "the epidemiology of mortality rates clearly indicates that the negative health outcomes beginning in early adolescence persist throughout the fourth decade of life" (1993, 8). William Gardner explains that only when we are older do the costs of taking risks outweigh the benefits. Income, for example, rises with age; so does our ability to predict the future: "A focus on the immediate rather than the long term consequences of a decision is a rational response to uncertainty about the future" (1993, 77). Perhaps to support our self-esteem as adults, we conveniently deny the frequency with which we act as adolescents are stereotypically thought to do, because we don't want to undermine our claims to status or damage our self-esteem (cf. Weinstein 1989).

10. Weinstein (1987) specifically links defensive denial with the notion of perceived seriousness, asserting that the emotion defended against is the fear of contracting the serious condition. Since perceived seriousness is negatively correlated with optimistic bias, Weinstein dismisses the role of defensive denial out-of-hand. However, if we define defensive denial more broadly, allowing it to include the defense of one's status and self-esteem, for example, then the emotions defended against include shame and embarrassment, the occurrence of which would be positively correlated with perceived preventability and so with optimistic bias according to Weinstein's own work (1987, 491). Accordingly, my use of the term "denial" in tandem with the term "optimistic bias" is appropriate.

11. Some of these women may have been consciously aware of their risks but wary of indicating them on the questionnaires, so the number of truly unaware women may actually be less than 70 percent. Nonetheless, biases affecting questionnaire responses about AIDS risk include those that affect risk perception itself. The point that risk perceptions are biased remains intact despite the figure's possible skew.

12. This idea was invoked by Steve Cokely, an aide to Chicago's mayor, in his public claim that Jewish doctors were injecting Black babies with HIV. This is not the only anti-Semitic rumor popular among certain segments of the Black community (cf. Turner 1993, 154). Black anti-Semitism also appears in the efforts of some to link Israel (in partnership with South Africa) with the invention of HIV (Secter 1988).

13. Sci.med.aids is a USENET newsgroup that discusses AIDS and HIV. According to its November 1993 statement of purpose, users and readers (numbering about 40,000) include people with HIV infections or AIDS, scientific researchers and authors, public health officials, AIDS service providers, educators and researchers, and other interested individuals. Topics include the causes of AIDS and opportunistic infections, vaccine for AIDS, treatment or cures for AIDS and opportunistic infections, and AIDS prevention and education. Sci.med.aids can be received as electronic mail through listserv@rutvml.rutgers.edu.

14. "Mr. Green" is a pseudonym. Hard copies of a number of his messages are in my files.

15. In her report on AIDS and genocide Guinan (1993) refers to a series of stories in the *Los Angeles Centennial.* Finding no record of a newspaper under that name, I can only guess that she means the *Sentinel.*

16. Several polls carried out by the popular press also support this contention. A 1990 *New York Times*/WCBS TV poll (*New York Times* 1992) found that 10 percent of Blacks believed absolutely that HIV was deliberately created to infect Blacks, and another 20 percent believed that this was possible. A Gallup/*Newsweek* poll cited by the *New York Times* (1992) produced similar results.

17. See previous note.

18. Here I must note that distrust is far from nonexistent among whites. Over half of the white participants in Herek and Capitanio's (1994) research voiced some distrust of experts (e.g., doctors, scientists, government officials). Whites were most likely to agree that information is being held back, and least likely to agree that AIDS is part of a genocidal plan.

19. Except where otherwise noted, information for this section was assembled largely from Weiss (1994) and the sci.med.aids "FAQ," a constantly updated article that sci.med.aids organizers post monthly to answer "frequently asked questions" about AIDS (see note 13).

20. According to Bates (1990) Strecker cites a 1972 issue of the *Bulletin of the*

World Health Organization (vol. 47, 259) which contains a request for a virus that harms the immune system. As Bates further notes, the July 1, 1969 issue of the *Congressional Record* contains evidence of a possible government-sponsored project aimed at creating a "synthetic biological agent . . . for which no natural immunity could have been acquired" (129).

21. There also has been much talk of HIV being spread through the oral polio vaccines administered in Central Africa in the 1950s and 1960s, thanks partly to the publicization of this theory in an article featured in *Rolling Stone* (Curtis 1992). Basically, some argue that because the vaccines were created with the use of monkey kidneys, SIV contamination — and so HIV contamination — could have occurred. *Rolling Stone* declared in an "update" that a committee of six "eminent scientists" convened expressly to investigate these charges concluded that this most probably did not happen (*Rolling Stone* 1993). While the suggestion that the polio vaccinations led to AIDS did not originate as a genocide theory (the alleged contamination was deemed accidental), it has been refashioned and appropriated by many genocidal thinkers, just as Strecker's theories have been.

22. Bates (1990) reports that this idea was developed with Strecker's assistance by dermatologist Alan Cantwell, Jr. in his book *AIDS and the Doctors of Death*. Strecker's theories, outlined in a 1986 letter to the editor of the *Journal of the Royal Society of Medicine* (Strecker 1986), are apparently detailed in a speech made in 1990 called "Is AIDS Man Made?" and in a video marketed by the Strecker Group called "The Strecker Memorandum."

23. While the Tuskegee Study's termination recently had its twentieth anniversary and received some media coverage, knowledge of the study — or at least of its details — may actually be limited to more educated and older citizens.

24. The Tuskegee Syphilis Study was originally planned to be cross-sectional; it was to be a single, time-limited effort in which researchers would examine men in various stages of the disease to ascertain the damage it could theoretically inflict on a (male) body over time. The original recruits received the then-standard heavy metals therapy involving mercury and arsenicals. It was later decided to turn the study into a long-term effort aimed at documenting the natural history of untreated syphilis. The men therefore did not receive antibiotic therapy when it became available in the 1940s. The original heavy metals treatments were conveniently forgotten by those who wrote the research reports submitted to medical journals (Edgar 1992).

25. The challenges of Black manhood are probably related to Farrakhan's alleged suggestion that a substance in the pituitary gland of the adolescent Black male will cure AIDS.

Chapter 4
Seropositivity Self-Disclosure and Concealment

People who have tested negative for HIV or who have not been tested at all often fear being lied to or manipulated by unethical seropositive individuals. This fear, in turn, affects risk-related behavior. Urban legends abound warning of beautiful HIV-positive charmers who enchant and then have unprotected sex with unsuspecting seronegative[1] people in order to spread the virus (regarding the social construction of AIDS and the further ramifications of myths such as this one, see Abelove 1994; cf. Farmer 1992; Turner 1993). Moreover, several cases in which HIV-positive individuals had unprotected sex with others while concealing their seropositivity have received extensive publicity.

Take, for example, the story of Gaetan Dugas, or "Patient Zero." Ralph Bolton notes that after the 1987 publication of Randy Shilts's *And the Band Played On*, which chronicled not only Dugas's progression from HIV infection to death but also his plenteous sexual liaisons, Dugas's story "was given extensive coverage and the role of his sexual escapades in spreading AIDS around the continent was highlighted" (1992, 20). Dugas was vilified despite the fact that he could not have known as we do today the role of sexual intercourse in HIV transmission — and despite the essential part he played in helping epidemiologists to describe that role. Bolton also describes the case of HIV-positive prostitute Fabian Bridges, who allegedly intentionally infected his clients. Bolton points out, "In both of these cases the promiscuous individual was blamed for continuing to have sex knowingly and intentionally without concern for the consequences to his partners, thereby linking promiscuity with psychopathology (Bersani 1988) and sickness with crime (Quam 1990, 34)" (1992, 20; citations in original).

Data from the few existing studies on HIV self-disclosure suggest that non-disclosure is indeed a problem. However, rather than hate and sinfulness, as implied in media reports such as those mentioned and in rumors of desperadoes who roam the streets at night spreading "the AIDS virus," non-disclosure may in many cases be motivated by loving intentions and a desire for intimacy (a motivation I return to in Chapter 9).

The Psychological Effects of Seropositivity

HIV test results generally take one to two weeks to be processed. The period between having one's blood drawn and finding out if one is or is not HIV positive can be trying (regarding the initial decision to get tested and the pros and cons of testing itself, see Bor et al. 1991; Coates et al. 1988; Meadows et al. 1990; see also Chapter 8). Many test-takers do not return to the test site to find out their results. Those who do return often find the clinicians' vocabulary for discussing the test confusing — and confusion can lead to mistaken interpretations of results. For instance, tested individuals sometimes interpret negative results as "bad" and as signifying infection, similarly, they may interpret positive results as "good" and as indicating that one is free of HIV. Further, as Kurth and Hutchison point out, people who think they have "passed" the HIV test sometimes equate their perceived negativity with immunity, which can lead to complacency or even an increase in high-risk behavior (1989; cf. Kinsey 1994).

In the case of positive test results, the testee must adjust to his or her new status as a person living with HIV (or, if the virus has progressed far enough, as a person living with AIDS — a PWA). Information on HIV and AIDS coping or adjustment processes is still limited. Most research concerns homosexual or bisexual urban men, who differ significantly from heterosexually oriented inner-city women not only in the obvious realms of gender, sexual orientation, and income, but also in social organization. (The relative strength of social networks in male homosexual communities, which rapidly mobilized upon recognition of the AIDS threat, has already been mentioned.)

As Norris Lang (1991) explains, while many aspects of an individual's identity come into play in the coping process, the homosexual man's responses to an HIV or AIDS diagnosis "appear to be related to the prior social and psychological adjustment of the gay male to his sexual orientation" (67). Those individuals who are "more constructive in this adjustment" (67) — those who are neither closeted nor guilt-ridden — deal better with seropositivity than those who deny their sexual orientation or preference.

Lang's report suggests that coping strategies or styles and personal biography or identity constructions play key roles in mediating how people deal with HIV seropositivity. Indeed, after studying the personal narratives of seropositive homosexual young men, William Borden found that "HIV seropositivity is likely to threaten existing interpretations of self, others, life experience, and anticipated future" (1991, 438); a positive HIV test may require a revision of one's life history, which can be devastating. As chapter 7 will show, untested and seronegative women generally believe in their own wisdom and skill in choosing safe partners, and they generally trust their partners' claims of fidelity. Conversely, after receiving seropositive test results, inner-city women talk of betrayal, broken trust, and partners who must not have really loved them (Ward 1993b).

Coping with HIV infection or a diagnosis of AIDS involves more than just reinterpreting the events of one's life. It also involves grieving for and ultimately accepting the loss of one's future, and adjusting, in some cases, to a partner's treachery and deceit. Furthermore, deaths from AIDS often are multiple, especially in hard-hit communities such as those in the inner cities, and they can have social as well as physical consequences. So even those seropositive people who do not experience abandonment by other seropositive people who die will surely face the experience of being abandoned by and so losing relationships with seronegative (or untested and presumably seronegative) people who desert. That experts still know relatively little about AIDS (although great progress has been made in a short time) makes positive HIV diagnoses even more awful, as does the stigma of the disease and the intense social and moral confusion that surround it (Earl et al. 1991–92).

Working with men, McCain and Gramling (1992) identified three separate phases of the process of coping with seropositivity and AIDS. These processual phases were (a) Living with Dying, (b) Fighting the Sickness, and (c) Getting Worn Out. "Living with Dying" begins with a positive diagnosis and the initial desire to deny it—a desire participants in McCain and Gramling's study were consciously aware of (cf. Earl et al. 1991–92). The desire is not limited to men: denial and related behaviors such as increased drug use are especially likely among substance-using women (Kurth and Hutchison 1989).

Beyond the urge to deny one's seropositive status—an urge that may be dodged or succumbed to—"Living with Dying" also entails "anger, depression, suicidal ideation, and fear of rejection by others" (McCain and Gramling 1992, 276). Sleep and communication disorders, increased anxiety, and hypochondria also have been observed during this phase. Both men and women seem to experience all these symptoms; and Kline et al. (1992) report that seropositivity in poor urban minority women has a negative effect on sexual interest levels, perhaps due to the women's fear of transmitting HIV to lovers.

Women also may feel overcome by guilt about their possible roles as transmitters of HIV to their children (HIV-positive women's reproductive options are discussed in Chapters 2 and 8). Women are probably as likely as closeted or homophobic homosexual men to "experience feelings of overwhelming shame" (Kurth and Hutchison 1989, 262) as a result of seropositivity, because it signals their participation in socially unacceptable practices (e.g., illicit drug use, multiple casual sexual relations, a relationship with a man who is unfaithful). It also may imply they are contaminated and contaminating. So stigmatized, HIV-positive women may feel unable to inform members of their social networks of their condition. This can lead to "increased isolation during a time of great need" (262).

Moving from the anger and fear of the first phase of coping into the next, "Fighting the Sickness," involves deciding, as McCain and Gramling say, to "get on with one's life" (1992, 278). Social network membership shifts as rejecting individuals drop out, as those deemed somehow threatening (e.g., as hateful, accusing, or merely unsupportive) are avoided, and as more HIV-positive individuals are incorporated (Barbara Limandri uses the word "colonizing" to describe the latter process, in which people with similar conditions seek one another out [1989, 77]). People "Fighting the Sickness" focus on maintaining their health, not just by locating and cultivating friendships with supportive people, but also by getting enough rest and eating properly. They become concerned with maintaining their weight and physical appearance.

While "Fighting the Sickness" often involves intentionally optimistic changes in mental attitude, one's financial and other resources come into play as well. Inner-city women who would like to nurture themselves often cannot because of material and social obstacles such as money shortages, familial responsibilities, and the classism, sexism, and racism built into the health care delivery system (see Chapter 2; see also Ward 1993a). Furthermore, inner-city women often are not diagnosed until AIDS has overtaken them (Kurth and Hutchison 1989). It is quite possible that they move through the second phase more quickly than homosexual men, if they even enter it before proceeding into the final stage, in which death is no longer fought. Alternatively, inner-city women's second coping phase may entail a completely different set of responses than it does for homosexual men.

Denial

Many people react initially to seropositivity with denial or disbelief; for some, this persists even as symptoms of AIDS develop (Earl et al. 1991–92). Denial seems counter-productive to outside observers for a variety of reasons. It is true that it is correlated with higher levels of sexual risk taking (e.g., Joseph et al. 1989). But, as Joseph et al. point out, "There is a

growing appreciation for the role of denial or illusion in the mainte-
nance of psychological functioning" (211). Chapter 7 will examine denial's effect on what Joseph et al. call "a robust sense of psychological
well-being" (211). Here, I simply wish to draw attention to their finding
that those who deny their seropositivity have lower (healthier, better)
emotional stress levels than those who do not deny their diagnoses.

Self-Disclosure

The Self-Disclosure Process

One of the challenges newly diagnosed HIV-positive individuals or PWAs
face is disclosing their status to others. While to the seronegative and to
the untested self-disclosure seems an imperative and obvious step, the
seropositive weigh a number of factors to determine whether and to
whom they will disclose. Existing data suggest that these factors include
fear of rejection, worry about the discreetness of the people disclosed to,
and shame for having a stigmatized condition. Self-disclosure can involve
revealing damning (culturally unacceptable) information about one's
conjugal relations (or one's drug use patterns) and this can be degrad-
ing. It also can entail having to face facts about oneself (or one's partner,
and one's relationship) that were more comfortable unacknowledged.
The disclosee could very well decide to abandon the self-discloser and
could tell others of his or her infection, as if sounding a warning. All of
this can have disastrous effects on the self-disclosing person.

Because self-disclosure is so potentially dangerous, deciding when and
if to do it is a complex matter. In a study of self-disclosure of a number of
stigmatizing conditions including HIV seropositivity, Barbara Limandri
(1989) found that episodes of self-disclosure can follow several patterns.
The disclosee's perceived responses to the information disclosed and to
the self-discloser are crucial. Sometimes, especially when knowing one's
serostatus causes great stress, self-disclosure can be venting (i.e., compulsive or explosive). Generally, however, self-disclosers "conceal for
awhile, disclose, then retract back into concealment" (73), searching for
signs that full revelation will not result in rejection. Disclosure then can
be reciprocal, facilitated when the disclosee chooses to reciprocate with
some kind of self-disclosure in return, or invitational, when the self-
discloser provides clues, inviting the disclosee to make inquiries.

Partner Notification or Third Party Disclosure

The kind of relationship the potential self-discloser has with the potential
disclosee (employee-boss, father-son, sister-brother, spouse) is an impor-

tant variable in the self-disclosure situation. Much of what we know about self-disclosure specifically to lovers comes from studies of partner notification or third party disclosure programs. These programs, through which third parties such as public health officials notify seropositive individuals' partners, free seropositive people from the burden of having to share their news, but also compromise their privacy.

Some research indicates that third party disclosure is successful if measured in economic terms. In a study of CDC-funded counseling, testing, referral, and partner notification (CTRPN) programs, Holtgrave et al. found that, despite the fact that HIV's long incubation period can make identifying and locating exposed individuals extremely difficult, "for every 100 HIV-seropositive persons identified and reached by CTRPN services, at least 20 new HIV infections are averted" (1993, 1225). Based on calculations of the lifetime treatment cost per seropositive patient, "the CDC's expenditure on HIV CTRPN services results in a substantial net economic benefit to society" (1229).

Partner notification programs offer another benefit besides the economic one: they offer a way to identify the possibility of infection in people (partners and ex-partners) who might not otherwise suspect it. As a *Lancet* editorial proclaimed, "Not offering a system of notification deprives at-risk individuals of the opportunity to get tested, seek medical care, and protect their contacts" (1991, 1113). The original seropositive individual's privacy need not be compromised if his or her name is not mentioned. Still, as Giesecke et al. argue, "Without guarantees of good medical and psychosocial care and support for diagnosed patients as well as of total confidentiality, a partner notification programme cannot be justified" (1991, 1097). Identifying seropositive individuals, affecting their health positively, and stemming HIV transmission are three different issues; the former goal need not entail the latter two, although, Giesecke et al. argue, it should.

In any case, note Giesecke et al. (1991), partner notification programs can be more effective than large-scale screening efforts at identifying HIV-positive individuals. They also might be more effective than self-disclosure. To test this, Landis et al. (1992) carried out a study in which mostly male, mostly Black, and mostly homosexual or bisexual HIV-positive individuals were randomly assigned to either a "patient-referral group" — a group in which participants were made responsible for informing their partners of their seropositivity — or a "provider-referral group" — a group in which a study counselor notified the partners. The partners to be notified included all people with whom each study participant had sex during the previous year. While the "provider-referral group" succeeded in notifying 50 percent of the partners, members of the "patient-referral group" only notified 7 percent. Landis et al. concluded that leaving notification up to seropositive individuals is "quite ineffective" (p. 101).

Self-Disclosure Research

The amount of research focused specifically on self-disclosure (as opposed to disclosure made by a third party) is negligible. While a few scholars have investigated intentions to self-disclose (e.g., Kegeles et al. 1988) and some individual case studies of non-disclosure have been documented (e.g., Chiodo and Tolle 1992), most of the available literature, limited as it is, takes the form of guidelines for HIV/AIDS counselors (e.g., Green 1989). The advice offered is generally impressionistic and suggestive, and although it may be useful to counselors, it is not research-based.[2] Results from only four actual studies on self-disclosure practices have been published. All four studies (to be described shortly) focus on homosexual and bisexual men.[3]

In addition to the papers regarding these four studies, there are publications in which self-disclosure to lovers is mentioned, but generally this is in passing. For example, McKeganey and Barnard (1992) devote a few pages of their book on injecting drug users (IDUs) and AIDS to a few participants' comments on the issue. McKeganey and Barnard seek to illuminate what it is like to be HIV positive and to show that seropositive people and IDUs in general are neither abnormal nor dangerous. But most other authors' references to self-disclosure to lovers are much less considered. For example, in concluding their report on risk reduction among HIV-positive women, Kline and VanLandingham mention that "anecdotal evidence suggests that in several cases women failed to disclose their serostatus to their partners" (1994, 401). The extent of non-disclosure and its effects on risk reduction are left unexamined. This is particularly notable because partner-related factors were ostensibly a main focus of the study.[4]

Pivnick (1993) also touches on non-disclosure to partners. Although she did not set out to study seropositivity self-disclosure (but rather the meaning of condoms among women attending a methadone clinic), she does note that her participant roster included sixteen married seropositive women. Fourteen of the sixteen had told their partners about their conditions. Interestingly, the two who had not self-disclosed insisted that their partners use condoms with them, but rather than tell their partners that this was because of HIV, both told them that the condoms were for contraception (436–38; this practice is explored further in Chapter 9).

As Table 1 shows, the proportion of methadone clinic women who self-disclosed is quite similar to the proportion of self-disclosers found in the four studies mentioned above (note that study methods differ and

TABLE 1. Serostatus Self-Disclosure Frequencies

Self-disclosure to primary partners

Hays et al. (1993)	98%
Marks et al. (1992a,b)	69%
Perry et al. (1994)	77%
Pivnick (1993)	88%
Schnell (1992)	89%

Self-disclosure to secondary partners

Marks et al. (1992a,b)	36%
Perry et al. (1994)	42%–47%

frequencies provided are not directly comparable). All five proportions seem on first glance to differ significantly from the previously noted "patient-referral group" findings of Landis et al. (1992), in which only 7 percent of HIV-positive individuals self-disclosed to partners.

For instance, in their study of mostly white, mostly educated, mostly well-off homosexual San Francisco men, Hays et al. (1993) found that, although asymptomatic men were less likely than symptomatic men to disclose their seropositivity to relatives and colleagues, virtually all of the men (98%) told their partners of their conditions. Similarly, using data from mostly white homosexual and bisexual men recruited in Dallas, Denver, Seattle, and Long Beach (CA), Schnell (1992) found a self-disclosure-to-partners rate of 89 percent. However, neither study explored self-disclosure to secondary or casual partners; the other two studies did.

In the third study, carried out with lower-income men from Los Angeles, most of whom were Hispanic and homosexual or bisexual, Marks et al. (Marks, Richardson, and Maldonado 1991; Marks, Richardson, Ruiz, et al. 1992a; Marks, Bundek, Richardson, et al. 1992b) found that subjects favored self-disclosure to partners known as seropositive (Marks, Richardson, and Maldonado 1991, 1322; cf. Hays et al. 1993 regarding the impact of a potential disclosee's sexual orientation on self-disclosure). Moreover, the likelihood of self-disclosure decreased as the number of partners in the previous year increased. This helps explain the 7 percent reported in Landis et al. (1992; see above), as that self-disclosure frequency includes a year's worth of both secondary as well as primary partners.

After summing the total number of partners mentioned by each participant, Marks et al. concluded that only one in twenty (5.5%) were notified (Marks, Richardson, Ruiz, et al. 1992, 102). However, more than two in three (69%) men with one partner had self-disclosed, as had more than one in three (36%) of those men with two to four partners. The pattern of results "remained virtually unchanged" after the few hetero-sexual and non-Hispanic men were excluded from analyses (Marks, Bundek, Richardson, et al. 1992, 302), suggesting that there is at least some room for generalizing from these studies to non-homosexually-oriented people and to non-Hispanics.

The fourth study, carried out by Perry et al. (1994; see also Perry et al. 1990) as part of a larger, ongoing project with mostly white homosexual men of mixed incomes, sought to clarify the relationship between self-disclosure to partners and social support, emotional distress, and physical distress. Most participants had multiple sex partners and were sexually active. Findings suggest that the participants who were least likely to inform sexual partners about their seropositivity had lower perceived levels of social support, no spouses or live-in partners, and felt less comfortable about their homosexual orientation.

Overall, after a mean of just over two (2.3) years since initial notification of seropositive status, 86 percent of the participants in the Perry et al. study (1994) had informed at least one sex partner, present or past, primary or casual.[5] Participants were more likely to have informed primary ("steady") sex partners, past or present, than they were to inform casual partners. The frequency with which present primary partners were informed was 77 percent, while 70 percent of past primary partners were informed. For casual partners, the percentages were 42 (present) and 47 (past). Although 14 percent of the participants did not self-disclose to any partner at all, overall rates of unsafe sex were low.

In summary, as Table 1 shows, the existing data on self-disclosure to partners suggest that the majority of seropositive people may tell their primary partners about their seropositivity. But not all will do so and, moreover, many do not tell past or secondary partners about their health conditions. There is then some basis to the fear that some seronegative (or untested) people harbor of having such information withheld, especially by a new or one-time partner.

Concealing one's positive serostatus undercuts partners' efforts to make informed decisions regarding safer sex. As Shtarkshall and Awerbuch point out, "Were the aware [seropositive] partner to disclose the relevant information, the unaware partner would be able to use the knowledge to assess his/her real risk of becoming infected" (1992, 124). Given the right conditions, the newly aware partner might approach sex more cautiously.[6] Of course, people cannot actually compute their "real" risk levels; the calculations are too complex. Nonetheless, non-awareness of partner seropositivity seems to be correlated with people's underestimation of their AIDS risk levels (p. 124).

Non-Disclosure

For non-disclosure as for self-disclosure to partners, few data exist; again, the research that has been done focuses on the experiences of men who have sex with men. The questionnaire used for the aforementioned study of mostly white, mostly educated, mostly well-off homosexual San Francisco men (Hays et al. 1993) included an open-ended question regarding the decision to keep one's seropositivity secret. The study concerned disclosure to parents, friends, coworkers, clinicians, landlords, and others as well as to primary partners. Many of the men decided not to disclose to certain people because they saw no benefit in doing so or because they felt that the costs would outweigh the benefits. Potential interpersonal costs included losing or damaging a relationship, causing another person undue stress, and having to deal with that person's emotional reactions to the news. The men also expressed concerns over revealing homosexuality as well as over the possibility of the disclosee's verbal indiscretion.

Desires for intimacy, continued love, and smooth relations seem to play a large part in motivating non-disclosure. So may a desire for safety: numerous women have been badly injured by partners after self-disclosing (e.g., *Baltimore Sun* 1993). Abandonment by an individual disclosed to also can threaten the self-discloser's physical well-being, as when she or he has been living with or supported by that person. Moreover, self-disclosure can lead to job termination, housing discrimination, and other practical problems.

Malicious Non-Disclosure

Psychological research indicates that upon seropositive diagnoses many people become angry; indeed, the first phase of coping with AIDS involves anger (McCain and Gramling 1992). Fury and rage may turn a person rancorous and vindictive. And when one does not know against whom to seek revenge — and in the case of AIDS it is frequently difficult to track down one's infector — any human target may do. But generally, anger subsides and people move on to enter stage two of the coping process, which involves fighting AIDS, not other people.

Still, rumors of vindictive people who slither through town spreading HIV among unknowing "victims" get passed around. Such rumors appeal to many individuals because, faced with the uncontrollable likes of the AIDS pandemic, our urges to attribute blame, to scapegoat run high. I discussed this in Chapter 3 in relation to racial or ethnic tension and defensive conspiratorial thought. Malicious non-disclosure differs from conspiratorial plotting in that individuals rather than highly organized

groups of confederates are the parties lurking, ready to entrap the un-
wary. In any case, people feel defenseless against non-disclosers. A metaphoric connection with the murderous and apparently conniving modus
operandi of the AIDS virus itself, for which there is no cure, comes to
mind.

All states have laws regarding seropositivity disclosure, but purposeful
non-disclosure is legally a shadowy area. Currently, a move is on to crim-
inalize intentional HIV transmission. Twenty-five states have criminal
transmission laws on the books (*Nation's Health* 1993). While essentially
everyone would agree that intentionally inflicting harm and conspiring
to murder someone (albeit slowly and torturously, as would be the case
with AIDS) is wrong, criminalization may not be the way to stop such
action. This is because criminal transmission laws may also be used in
selective scapegoating. In fact, according to an editorial in *Nation's Health*
(1993), criminal transmission laws are commonly used against prostitutes
and prisoners.

Wrongful accusations are sure to accompany the prejudicial applica-
tion of criminal transmission laws. For example, a seropositive individual
who develops a nose bleed while sitting in a hospital waiting room and
who then accidentally trips on the way to the front desk for tissues and
assistance, thereby unintentionally splattering blood droplets over several people, may be charged with recklessly and purposefully endanger-
ing the lives of others. How is this individual to prove his or her inno-
cence? Intentions are perhaps harder to discern when the sexual arena
serves as the site of potential transmission. The emotions surrounding
sexual events (especially taboo ones) often run higher than those surrounding other kinds of social interactions, making the pursuit of truth
even more challenging.

The stigma AIDS carries and the emotions it triggers make criminalization a dangerous step not only because it will lead to scapegoating and
frame-ups, but also because it legitimizes extrapunitive or attributional
thinking regarding the vectors of infection and the efficacy of taking self-
protective measures. That is, criminalization encourages people to think
about HIV as something that others infect them with and so as a threat
that they can do nothing about.

In regard to a case being tried in Illinois at the end of 1993 (*Nation's
Health* 1993), the American Public Health Association and the Illinois
Public Health Association declared in court that criminalization generates panic and fear. Criminalization may stop people from seeking testing
and counseling because of a fear that law enforcement officials may ob-
tain test results. Furthermore, a non-disclosing seropositive person's dili-
gent condom use during sex may not be a defense under some laws
because condoms are not 100 percent effective, and media coverage of

this may "create dangerous confusion in a public in dire need of clear educational messages on condom use." Both associations argued that criminalization threatens to undermine public health efforts to combat AIDS.

The threat of HIV infection has generated many responses, some hysterical, some level-headed, and some apathetic. This and the preceding chapters have examined many of these reactions and summarized the various experiences that accompany seropositivity. Having introduced the reader to AIDS, and having reviewed the relevant literature on education and AIDS-risk perception, I turn to my research. The next four chapters describe work on AIDS-risk denial among inner-city women. They will show that unsafe sex has psychosocial benefits that, in the short run, make it an appealing plan of action for women, who strategically use unsafe sex to gain many of the social and emotional resources that they need from men.

Notes

1. Many people assumed to be seronegative actually have not been tested. This fact should be borne in mind as the reader considers sex between a seropositive person and any other individual who has not explicitly tested positive for HIV antibodies.

2. Some advice to counselors is research based, but the research it is based on has generally been undertaken in regard to chronic diseases or conditions other than AIDS.

3. Unpublished results from research carried out with a small sample of seropositive women (N = 25) by Chervenak and Weiss (as cited in Marks et al. 1991, 1321) show that over half (52%) had self-disclosed to their partners.

4. It may reflect a culturally encouraged tendency to assume that the HIV-positive individual's self-disclosure of serostatus automatically or "naturally" accompanies sexual interaction, as revealed in the investigators' choice of the phrase "failed to disclose" (Kline and VanLandingham 1994, 401).

5. Seventy-one percent of the participants had informed at least one present partner, and seventy percent had informed at least one past partner.

6. Perry et al. (1994, 1990) report that self-disclosure of positive serostatus is not associated with a greater likelihood of safer sex practices. The replicability of this important finding and the applicability it has for heterosexuals remains to be seen.

Chapter 5
The Condom Use Project

My original research mission involved investigating the low efficacy of AIDS education in Cleveland's M&I clinics in order to improve it. My main aims were to find out why most clients neglected to comply with the safer-sex guidelines provided, and to identify the factors distinguishing the non-users from the few who did use condoms.[1]

It is folly to believe that education alone can halt the spread of AIDS (see Chapter 3). The constraints that sexism, racism, and other oppressions place on people's perception of AIDS risks and on their abilities to reduce these risks are immense. Vast social, cultural, and economic changes need to be made if we are actually going to stem the pandemic. Accordingly, this research helps clarify the nature of the social and cultural changes needed to enable women to avoid unsafe sex, and enhances our understanding of the cultural constructions of love, relationships, and self-concept—constructions that have a great impact on the effects of AIDS education efforts.

The project was originally scheduled to last for one year. It used focus groups and interviews, and was funded by a grant from Cleveland's Community AIDS Partnership Project. Anticipating the importance of the findings, I applied to the Spring Foundation for Research on Women in Contemporary Society for a second grant. A second phase was initiated; this time questionnaires and interviews were used. All told, about 150 women participated in the research. Here I should note that, while AIDS is a growing problem among teens, legal and logistical considerations led me to limit this study to adults; that is, women under eighteen years of age were prohibited from participating. Age averages should be interpreted with this in mind.

The focus group discussions and preliminary interviews guided me to many of the AIDS-related themes most salient for the women, and the use of questionnaires enabled the collection of quantitative data. The final set of interviews provided the rich first-person narratives that form the heart of this book's message. The data are presented in the chapters that follow. Here, I describe the setting and methods in detail.

Cleveland, Ohio

Cleveland is a mid-sized city of about half a million people located where the Cuyahoga River meets the southern shore of Lake Erie. Stretching along the lake's shore and divided by the river into east and west sides, Cleveland was once a great hub of industrial, mercantile, and shipping activity. This was partly due to the easy access the city had to coal and iron ore.

Until World War I, most of the people who had settled in Cleveland came from the Eastern United States or from Europe. But a labor shortage in 1918 brought many Blacks from the Southeast and many whites from Appalachia up to the city. After World War II, newcomers to the city's center, much of which is now on the east side of the river, were mostly Black. Unfortunately, many of these newcomers did not have the specialized skills then necessary for factory employment. Furthermore, as production techniques and products themselves changed, industry abandoned the center of the city for the suburbs. Middle-class people followed. On the east side, the resulting concentration of inner-city Blacks living in poverty and subject to its accompanying pressures contributed to serious rioting in 1966.[2]

By 1990, the city's population, which in 1940 was nearly 900,000, had dropped to just over 500,000 (CUPSC 1992). The glory of Cleveland's past and the possibilities its future holds notwithstanding, its inner city has suffered the fate most Northeastern inner cities have suffered. While some banks, big hotels, restaurants, bars, and fortified shopping malls still call a half-dozen square downtown blocks home, and while gentrification has added to property values in certain urban pockets, the holdouts are ringed by a wide arc of destitution. In 1990, 29 percent of Cleveland's residents lived in poverty (CUPSC 1992). Driving between the downtown area and my office at Case Western Reserve University, which sits on the eastern edge of the city, I would pass many boarded-up businesses, run-down wood-frame houses, and empty lots. People advised me to keep my car doors locked when traversing this burned-out area. If I was foolish enough to drive downtown at night, I should not stop even for red lights, they said.

Just past the university, the city gives way to the suburbs, where flight took most east-side whites and where similar class and safety concerns took most of the city's more prosperous Blacks. While Blacks and whites do interact to some degree in the suburbs, Black and white residents of

Cleveland proper have extremely low chances of dealing with each other and they rarely live in the same neighborhoods. By these criteria, Cleveland is the nation's second most segregated city (Chicago is the first; Massey and Denton 1988).

Public health clinics and social welfare centers are scattered throughout the city's neighborhoods. The social welfare center where I conducted much of the preliminary research was south of the university, in a largely nonresidential area on the north edge of a neighborhood increasingly occupied by Jamaican and other West Indian immigrants with African heritage. The health center where I worked during the second phase of data collection was located north of the university, toward the lake, in a neighborhood I shall call North End. My mother's family lived in this neighborhood more than fifty years ago. She and her female kin would probably have sought health care in the very clinic where I conducted my fieldwork, had it existed then.

As the majority of the research participants were recruited at the health center in North End, a neighborhood sketch is appropriate here. About 26,000 people lived in North End in 1990, the last year for which neighborhood profile information (CUPSC 1992) is available; 98 percent of these people were Black. While women of childbearing age (between fifteen and forty-four years old) comprised 23 percent of North End's population, men of that age range accounted for only 19 percent of North End's residents.

About half of all household groups (48%) lived in rental units in 1990. Less than one in three households with children (30%) were headed by married couples; two in three (64%) were female headed; one in fourteen (7%) were male headed.[3] Exactly 850 in 1000 live births were to unwed mothers and about 10 percent of all teenage females had babies. The infant mortality rate was 26 per 1000 live births; the rate of low birth weights was 149 per 1000.

More than one in three (35%) of North End's residents lived in poverty. 48 percent received food stamps; about one in eight (12.4%) received Aid for Families with Dependent Children (AFDC); just less than one in nine (11.6%) received general assistance. The rate of drug violation arrests per 1000 residents was eighteen, and the crime rate (which reflects assault, aggravated assault, auto theft, burglary, larceny, homicide, rape, and robbery) was 112 per 1000.

Driving to the social welfare and health centers from the university, I passed numerous store-front churches, corner shops, and fast-food establishments; I also passed schools and well-used libraries. In winter, the emptiness of the streets, the omnipresent architectural decay, and the overall grayness and icy chill made the drive depressing. But the commute was a pleasure in spring and summer, when flowers blossomed, trees grew green, and the streets filled up with people of all ages going about the business of life.

Phase One: M&I Neighborhood Women

Focus Groups

In its first phase, the study used focus (discussion) groups and individual interviews. Medical anthropologists often use focus groups for rapid data collection when seeking answers to highly specific questions, dealing with severe health threats that demand immediate responses, and developing questionnaires and other data collection instruments such as interview schedules (Pelto and Pelto 1990). Several AIDS-related projects dealing with Black inner-city women already have used the focus group method; these and other sex-related projects show that women in focus groups can be "very open and uninhibited in discussing highly personal subject matters" (Shervington 1993; for examples see Flaskerud and Rush 1989; Fullilove et al. 1990; Worth 1989; see also Basch 1987). Institutional limitations made it impossible to hold focus groups at that time with M&I clinic clients, so participants were recruited through the aforementioned social welfare center, which serves women also served by the M&I clinics.

Instead of pulling together women who were strangers, I contacted a few of the social workers to ask about the possibility of securing the participation of several of the ongoing discussion groups that they oversaw. I did this because, in addition to being fairly representative of the M&I clients, the women in the groups would already have gotten to know one another and would be used to discussing personal issues in front of others, social workers and similar officials included (on this method of selection, see Bender and Ewbank 1994, cf. VanLandingham et al.; on the commonplace nature of open discussions related to sex in the Black community, see Fullilove et al. 1990). The members of the three parenting groups that were then in effect agreed to participate (these groups meet weekly to discuss childrearing problems). Confidentiality and anonymity was assured and written consent was received from each participant.

There were, on average, eight participants in each group (group turnout fluctuated slightly from week to week, and male partners sometimes attended; participants were used to this). Most were Black and all were poor. Those participants who had the emotional, social, and other resources needed to do so were working toward improving their own lives and broadening their children's opportunities. Twenty-three-year-old Clarissa, for example, who had a four-year-old daughter in her mother's care, attended the local junior college part-time. She wanted to go into teaching. Another group member, June, worked part-time looking after an elderly woman. She had just met a man whom she hoped to marry and the two were expecting a child. June regained custody of her eight-year-old son Gerald just after we finished the focus group sessions; he was in foster care because of June's (recently relinquished) crack-cocaine habit.

Meetings took place in a lounge on the top floor of the social welfare center, a rundown, boxy, three-story building located on a main thoroughfare. The building was one of many satellite buildings surrounding a large public hospital, forming a stony gray health-care complex that seemed to extend for blocks. There were no businesses close by and the area got very little foot-traffic. The focus groups were convened in winter; the bare trees and dirty patches of snow that framed the center heightened the bleakness of the research setting.

The lounge where groups met had windows looking down on the street and was furnished with two old sofas, a few old easy chairs, a Formica coffee table, a few end tables with ashtrays and thrift-shop lamps, and several institutional-style chairs with vinyl covered padding. While the lounge was being used for group sessions, people who had other business at the center met and chatted in the hallway outside the closed lounge door, or sat in the few chairs placed against the wall of a large open area a little further down the hall, where the secretarial staff did their work. They sometimes visited the small back room that was used for child care during group sessions as well as for housing donated clothing that clients could pick through.

Teams of two researchers supervised by Margaret Ruble visited each of the three participating groups four times.[4] Once a week for four weeks the assigned research teams introduced a variety of AIDS-related subjects according to a four-part topic schedule. Group members discussed the topics among themselves so that key dimensions of the intracultural debate surrounding AIDS could be studied and so that shared or intersubjectively held understandings could be documented (cf. Schwartz 1978). Researchers took notes and interrupted only to ask for clarifications of points made or words used, or to refocus the discussions. Many participants told us that they enjoyed the sessions and that they appreciated the value we placed on their opinions.

The first week, participants discussed their general beliefs about AIDS: what it is, where it came from, how it works. The second week, they concentrated on their beliefs about the costs and the benefits of both safer and unsafe sex. Discussion next focused on peoples' sense of vulnerability to AIDS, and participants finished up with a session on gender-linked considerations, such as heterosexual power dynamics.

Partly because of the topics and partly because of the tenor of the groups, language often was graphic and emotions overt. Personalities emerged almost immediately: Clarissa was prone to pouting (and others insulted her for this regularly), June liked pontificating, Elaine frequently referred to God, Jo told wonderfully ribald jokes about her and her husband's sex life, and Billie never said a word. Women sometimes talked over one another but they always agreed to clarify, elaborate, and re-capitulate for the researchers when this was deemed necessary.[5]

After concluding the four weeks of group discussion, an AIDS educa-tor from the M&I clinics visited each group. I arranged for this because AIDS-related projects provoke certain questions for participants; to leave these unanswered would be unethical. Also, staging an AIDS education session would allow us to gauge participants' response to the standard M&I curricula, which includes a video with several safer-sex scenarios and a lesson in transmission, time for questions, and free condoms (each M&I client is educated individually and first completes a survey which her educator uses as a guide, but participants did not do this). The research teams observed the reception that the education sessions re-ceived and asked for reactions later in one-on-one interviews, where we also followed up on the more salient issues raised in the discussions (see Spradley 1980 regarding feedback-driven research).

Interviews

Thirteen women from the focus groups were interviewed. We waited un-til after the series of discussions had been completed so that the women would be familiar with us; I expect that the accrued trust increased the validity of the data collected. Each interview followed a formal schedule, but interviewers' agendas remained flexible (see Spradley 1980) so that unanticipated information could be collected when it arose (cf. Dorfman et al. 1992). The interview schedule included forced-choice and open-ended questions. Several hypothetical scenarios (concerning situations such as a man and a woman meeting at a party and deciding to have sex) were also used to elicit information much the way projective tests do (cf. Abramson 1992). The interviews generally lasted for one and one-half hours. Again, informed written consent was secured. Interviewees were paid twenty-five dollars for their time and to cover their transportation.[6]

The fact that interviewees went through an AIDS education session and had been thinking about AIDS as a result of the project no doubt affected their interview responses. In order to do a rough check on the degrees and directions of their biases and to increase the interview sam-ple size, we also interviewed five female community members who did not participate in the discussions or in the educational segment.[7]

Phase Two: In The Clinic

Questionnaire

The focus group and interview data collected in phase one were analyzed and used to generate a questionnaire. The questionnaire, designed with the help of M&I clinicians Donna Dayse, Barbara Hood, and Deborah Washington, dealt with a broad range of AIDS-related topics but focused mainly on male economic contributions to the household and on women's extraconjugal social support systems. Because many clinic clients have low literacy skills, the questionnaire used simple language and mainly yes-no, other forced choice, and Likert-type scaled questions (i.e., questions with a range of answers, e.g., never, rarely, sometimes, often, very often, always).

Thirty pilot or pre-test questionnaires were administered to a convenience sample of thirty M&I clients waiting to be seen for pre- or post-natal care; consent was verbal and no names were taken. Each woman received five dollars. After reviewing the women's responses, I made some revisions to the questionnaire with Dayse's help; we then collected sixty revised questionnaires using the same methods as for the pilot version.[8] The few revisions made were mostly intended to increase the reliability and extensivity of the financial data collected. Basically, however, the questionnaires stayed the same. All in all, ninety were completed.[9]

As mentioned, the questionnaire focused mainly on economic and social network data. To identify the extent of male financial contributions to female households, participants were asked if they relied on anyone at all for money regularly; at a later point, the questionnaire asked if their partners were employed and if they ever received financial help from them. Participants also were asked to indicate on Likert-type scales how often their partners gave them certain kinds of non-monetary gifts (like food, clothing, small appliances, or help around the house), if at all.

To facilitate testing the hypothesis that unsafe sex and extraconjugal social support are linked, William Dressler's definition of "social support" as "the perceived availability of help or assistance from other persons during times of felt need" and his definition of a "social support system" as "a subset of an individual's ego-centered social network" (1991, 19) were followed. The extensivity of participants' extraconjugal support systems was ascertained by asking for a list of the individuals that each deemed important. Participants then were asked if they needed or wanted help with child care or housework, money, or advice, and if such help was forthcoming. Other questions determined how often the respondent relied on her social support network (if at all) and who provided the most help. Finally, participants were asked how often they felt "all alone in the world," with "no one to turn to for help." The questions measured how good each woman felt about different aspects of her social support network and how effective the network as a whole was for her.[10]

In addition to finances and networks, the questionnaire broached a few other topics. It included several questions about sexual practice and some about demographic details.[11] Data on women's attitudes toward and their histories of HIV testing were collected, and questions were asked about self-perceived risk factors, including whether or not one's partner had cheated or was cheating and what this meant to the respondent.

Interviews

After the questionnaires had been administered, a focus group was held at the clinic. Participants were given ten dollars each for their time. We told them about some of our preliminary findings and asked them to discuss the merit of these. Participants were also asked to tell us whatever they thought we should know regarding condom use and non-use among their peers. Their comments and the preliminary questionnaire and first-phase findings were used to design a final interview protocol.

The final interviews focused on women's extraconjugal support networks, the quality and style of their conjugal relations, and their financial situations. Several condom use and demographic questions were included. Each interview followed a formal questioning schedule but, as with the first set of interviews, the agenda remained flexible (see Spradley 1980) so that unanticipated information could be collected when it arose (cf. Dorfman et al. 1992).

The interviews took place in various private offices at the clinic and I conducted all of them. Generally, I would arrive at the clinic at nine, just after the morning rush of clients had been registered. After telling Dayse that I was there, I waited in the reception area, sometimes watching morning talk shows with the rest of the waiting clients. If few clients were present, I might talk with the receptionists about the clinic or the weather or somebody's upcoming vacation. The reception room, which was upstairs in a large, two-story building, housed a number of rotating clinics in addition to the M&I clinic, which had a semi-permanent allotment of the private consultation offices that lined its far side. There were about thirty plastic chairs; apart from the eight or so that lined the entry-side wall, most were arranged in four rows facing toward the television and away from the receptionists' desks.

Generally, apart from the occasional cockroach wending its way up a wall, there was little action in the waiting area. People sat quietly, looking at the television or talking softly. Occasionally, a crying baby would break the peace. Once, two men, who because of their attire seemed to be wards of the court fulfilling work orders, were brought in by a building supervisor to clean the floor. Another time, the M&I receptionist casually got herself a bucket of disinfectant and thoroughly cleaned the chair by her desk, which clients sit on as she updates their files and takes their blood pressure; one of the morning's clients had been diagnosed with a contagious topical infection.

Dayse approached adult clients whom she knew were in relationships, explained the study to them, and sought their participation for me. Consent was verbal and no names were taken. Each woman received twenty-five dollars for participating. Some days I would wait for a long time until an eligible woman was available, but other days I had to turn interested women away. If a woman agreed to participate (and all who were asked to did) then Dayse introduced her to me and helped us find an empty office to talk in. The interviews generally lasted for about one and one-quarter hours. I usually conducted two interviews each morning that I went to the clinic. After finishing, I would go downstairs, chat about baseball or the news headlines with the security guard, and walk to my car. Staff members always advised me to be careful on my way in and out of the building, as several muggings had recently taken place. I was advised to park my car within sight of the front door when possible.

Participants

The typical participant was about twenty-eight years old, Black, had completed the eleventh grade, and had two children.[12] While all the women lived impoverished inner-city lives, the majority had some sort of regular income. Over one-third were employed in the paid labor force (usually at menial part-time jobs); about half received welfare assistance; a few both had jobs and got assistance. Some participants made money by doing hair or nails for other women or by baby-sitting or cleaning houses; some reported receiving financial assistance from their male partners (about three-quarters of the women were in serious relationships[13]). Most had plans to better their lives, whether by attending nurse's aide certification classes or by saving money so that they and their children could move to a better apartment or duplex.

In the chapters to follow, I present a picture of what heterosexual relationships are like for these women. In general, focus group and questionnaire findings provide the basis for the broad statements I make and data from the final interviews provide specific illustrations (profiles of each of the clinic interviewees can be found in Appendix A). Although data were collected at two sites and from several subsets of women, such cross-referencing is justified by the similar backgrounds of the participants and by the fact that all of them are members of the group served by M&I clinics.

Here I should note that, while some of the women who completed the questionnaire were not in relationships, all interviewees were; interview data are used accordingly to avoid generating moot hypotheses. Also, as the focus of this book is ethnographic or qualitative, many of the quantitative data are presented in chapter notes or in Appendix B (to which I refer when relevant). I include in the text only raw numbers and some frequencies for making comparisons; because I used what might be called convenience samples, and because low condom use rates meant that the research included only small numbers of condom using women, including statistical test results as if they were meaningful would be inappropriate and irresponsible.

Generalizing from Study Results

Results from the study suggest that unsafe sex occurs most frequently among socially isolated women who derive self-esteem and status mainly from having conjugal partnerships with men. But because this project used small convenience-type samples of poor urban Blacks, the findings cannot be used to make scientifically valid generalizations regarding all U.S. Blacks; generalizations about women of other ethnicities, poor and urban or otherwise, are out of the question. However, findings from general health-risk perception and AIDS-risk perception research carried out with ethnically mixed groups show correspondences between the marriage and gender-related aspirations of women of color and those of mainstream U.S. women (e.g., Harrison et al. 1991; Kline et al. 1992; Prohaska et al. 1990; Sibthorpe 1992; Weinstein 1989, 1987; see also Carovano 1991).[14] These correspondences, and my own exploratory comparative work (see Preface), support my belief that the condom-use and other HIV/AIDS-related patterns and processes that I shall describe can also be found among white and perhaps other U.S. women as well. As the next chapters show, gender may well be more important than ethnicity and geography in the production of personal AIDS-risk denial.

Notes

1. I also wanted to test the feasibility of motivating women to practice safer sex by highlighting the threat that their own HIV seropositivity would have for their children, as an educational program involving this tactic was being considered.

2. The demographic composition of Cleveland's west side is different, with more poor whites and fewer poor Blacks. A small group of Hispanics, mostly of Puerto Rican descent, also live mostly on the west side of the river.

3. Of all households, 31 percent were comprised of unrelated individuals.

4. First phase data were collected by Sara Colegrove, Sandra Marchese, Candis Platt, Margaret Ruble, and myself; one of us is Black and four of us are white.

5. Although the focus of the study is qualitative, participants were asked to complete a short survey during the third week. Basic demographic data were collected this way; the survey also posed several questions about sexual practices, AIDS-related beliefs, and rates of safer sex that could only be answered privately for reasons concerning confidentiality. The group that I observed completed their surveys during the fourth week, as the discussion in week three was too intense to interrupt. Nineteen women completed the survey.

6. I donated the money set aside for focus group participant fees to the social welfare center, because the director felt that giving money to women who were there by court order (e.g., for neglecting their children) would be inappropriate and that it would be unfair to provide money to some clients (those in the participating parenting groups) but not to the rest.

7. Even though community interviewees were recruited by regular participants with whom they probably discussed the project, and although we spoke with only five of them, similarities and differences between their responses and those of the regular participants were attended to when interviews were analyzed.

8. Clinicians administered the questionnaire because their clients have not, historically, been comfortable or honest when answering questions for unknown outside researchers. However, I must acknowledge the possibility that, despite assurances of anonymity, some participants may have worried about clinician reactions and so may have given socially desirable rather than truthful responses to the questions asked.

9. Sixty-eight Blacks (75.6%), eighteen whites (20%), and four women of other ethnicities (4.4%) completed the questionnaire. The average respondent was almost twenty-six years old (adolescents were excluded for legal and logistical reasons). About two-thirds of the women were mothers; these women had about two children each. Educational data were not collected from the sixty women who completed the final questionnaire because the question asking for it had bothered some of thirty women who completed the pilot version; however, most of the original thirty women had finished the eleventh grade. While all re- spondents lived impoverished inner-city lives, seventy-five (83.3%) of the ninety women had regular incomes: thirty-eight (42.2%) participated in the paid labor force; thirty-six (40%) received public assistance; one woman (1.1%) reported both having a job and receiving assistance. Sixty-eight of the women (75.6%) had husbands or boyfriends, and fifty-eight of these involved women (85.3%) said that they loved their partners.

10. While the literature provided ideas about research directions, the specific- ity of existing measures for social support (Orth-Gomer and Unden 1987) led me to design my own such measure.

11. Phase one women were of the same socioeconomic and cultural back- ground and from the same neighborhoods as the M&I clients. Many have been or are clinic clients themselves, and I occasionally ran into them in the clinic during the second phase of data collection. They face similar daily challenges. However, as phase two unfolded I found that the first-phase women were, on average, about three years older than clinic clients. Also, some clinic clients were just beginning their reproductive careers. Further, almost all the first-phase participants have had the state intervene in their lives due to domestic troubles while many clinic clients have not been subjected to such.

12. There were slight differences between the samples of women involved in

the project's disparate phases. The typical phase one participant was about thirty years old, had completed the eleventh grade, and had two children. Almost half were employed, usually at menial part-time jobs; nearly all received welfare assistance. Some participants made money by doing hair or nails for other women; some reported receiving financial assistance from their male partners. The average phase-two interviewee was about twenty-eight years old, a high-school graduate, and a mother of two. One-third had jobs; two-thirds received public assistance. Questionnaire respondents are described in note nine (see also note 11).

13. The exception to this is found among second-phase interviewees, all of whom were partnered. This was so that the lack of condom use in long term or serious heterosexual relationships could better be explored.

14. While Blacks may favor marrying later than whites do and many condone single parenthood (Pittman et al. 1992), the two groups hold the same basic ideals for conjugal relations (e.g., Cochran 1989; Liebow 1967; Oliver 1989; Stack 1974). Anderson (1990) describes the ways mainstream American heterosexual ideals are promoted to Blacks, and he discusses Blacks' belief in "the dream" of achieving such relationships. He and the other authors cited describe and analyze the factors that keep many Blacks from actualizing these ideals as well as the ways that Blacks have responded to and compensated for having their conjugal goals obstructed.

Chapter 6
Romance and Finance

The common assumption that impoverished women engage in unprotected sex because of financial coercion and a lack of empowerment pervades a great deal of both popular and academic thinking about lower-income minority women and AIDS (cf. Kline et al. 1992; for examples of models that give economics a prime role see Carovano 1991; De La Cancela 1989; Ward 1993a; see also Campbell 1990; Worth 1989; regarding the political economy of STDs in general see Jones 1991). Deployed in certain contexts, assumption reveals and perpetuates racism and classism: it would never be used to explain sexual risk taking among white women belonging to the middle and upper classes. Politics notwithstanding, my research findings provide cause to question the assumed-to-be direct link between finance and romance. Findings suggest that inner-city women often have unsafe sex for reasons that have less to do with money per se than with the cultural ideals for heterosexual relationships and gender roles that certain political-economic conditions associated with capitalism help generate (regarding the latter, see Sobo n.d.). This is because these ideals leave most women who believe in them emotionally and socially dependent on relationships with men; accordingly, they affect women's perceptions of risk such that unsafe sex seems a safe bet (Sobo 1993a; cf. Kline et al. 1992).

Because materialist stereotypes are so pervasive, any discussion of women's social and emotional dependence on men must be preceded by an examination of the connection between money and love. Men's employment status and their attitudes about money do alter the ways that women evaluate them. But, as this chapter shows, most women do not perceive their own participation in condomless sex as purchased by men, nor do they generally see it as forced upon them by a need for men's money. Male cash aid to women in inner-city environments is unsteady at best. Further, the act of accepting resources from male sex partners can lead to exacerbated gender-related status inequities, which many women find unacceptable. This chapter examines these issues as it asks what exactly study women look for in men.

Money, Sex, and Love

As seen in Chapter 3, much of the literature on Black women's sexuality focuses on the economic and structural reasons for the alleged emphasis that Black women place on the instrumental dimension of sex. For example, it is thought that women must compete for men because they need men's money, and a willingness to have sex as men want it (without condoms) narrows the competition (e.g., Worth 1989). Furthermore, having children — which necessarily involves unprotected sex — can be cast (among other things) as economically desirable for women, whether in or out of wedlock, given the lack of alternatives or career opportunities (e.g., Mays and Cochran 1988). Having a baby can be a way of trying to establish social links with or through men. Moreover, having responsibilities to a child is often a prerequisite for membership in female support networks (e.g., Ward 1990).

While economic and structural factors do, no doubt, impact on sexuality, some of the data ushered to support materialist hypotheses actually can be seen to contradict and undermine them. For instance, to support the notion of female competition for male money it is often noted that a disproportionate number of Black males are unemployed, underemployed, or imprisoned (e.g., Oliver 1989; Worth 1989).[1] But many fail to note further that the poor state of most men's finances limits the material benefits women can gain from heterosexual relationships. Indeed, William Wilson (1987) explains that some Black women, knowing that the supply of employed men is small, choose to build families and network connections without the perceived burden of a husband or boyfriend. Pittman et al. point out that Black women are socialized to be economically independent, as does Pamela Wilson (1986). Kline et al. report, "Rather than occupying financially dependent roles in relationships with men, [poor urban] women [are] often forced to assume economic control" (1992, 450). Growing up, Black girls often learn early to assume adult responsibilities and they experience a more egalitarian family structure and have less traditional sex-role expectations than whites (Wingood and DiClemente 1992). And, as Weinberg and Williams (1988) note, women often provide male lovers with money rather than the other way around.

Nevertheless, the literature on Black sexuality generally ignores economic self-sufficiency among women when discussing behavior deemed by the mainstream as puzzling, deviant, or immoral (such as unsafe, premarital, or non-monogamous sex), preferring to ascribe such conduct to financial necessity.[2] Through a focus on neediness, scholars can provide women with apparently rational motives. In doing so they can adopt a seemingly non-judgmental stance: profit-seeking makes sense according to capitalist logic, and hunger can be used to excuse or explain moral breaches. I do not deny the force of financial need; however, simple cause-effect materialist models were not supported by my findings regarding the financial positions of the women.

The findings point to the importance of intervening psychocultural and social factors that, shaped as they are by larger political-economic forces, enable or inhibit the risk behaviors I examined. Admittedly, such factors are often introduced into materialist or socioeconomic arguments, where they provide a sense of contextual depth (e.g., De La Cancela 1989; Mays and Cochran 1988; Worth 1989); however, their introduction is sometimes perfunctory and, whether or not this is the case, often they are only superficially treated.[3]

One of the intervening factors mentioned most often is "self-efficacy" (the feeling that one can and will act on something; see Bandura 1977). Women's self-efficacy can be low as a result of their (financial) dependence on men and their perceptions about their options and about the power structure inherent in heterosexist conjugal relations. These perceptions condition decision making and affect sex-related communication. They decrease women's ability to avoid intercourse or to introduce innovations such as condom use (Copelon 1990; Muir 1991, 153; Schneider 1988).[4] Or, as I later explain, reality may be more psychoculturally complex.

Some of the models used to understand male sexual patterns are more sophisticated than those put forth for females in that they make fuller use of psychocultural and social factors. For instance, although the high level of non-monogamous heterosexual intercourse often achieved by Black men is frequently traced to their lack of economic opportunity, the latter is not said to generate sex for financial gain. Instead, it generates a culturally mediated dependence on favorable peer evaluations and a related tendency toward hyper-masculine behavior. In the place of career achievement for men, Black inner-city culture recommends sexual achievement, and so men build reputations through sexual conquest (Anderson 1990; Liebow 1967; Oliver 1989; Pittman et al. 1992; for statistics on non-monogamy[5] see Blumstein and Schwartz 1983, cited in Turner et al. 1989, 110–11[6]; also see Bower 1991, and Johnson 1993, 51–57).

Women who depend on men for money can indeed be forced by circumstance to ignore the infidelities of their male partners while engaging in what Marie Muir calls "survival sex" (1991, 153). However, taking cues from the above model of Black male sexuality as well as from the women about whom I write, I propose that while women often do get some money from men, something other than direct economic dependence (or related self-efficacy deficits) motivates them to have unsafe sex. The immediate reasons behind most women's unsafe sexual practices have to do with the culturally recommended strategies for garnering favorable peer- and self-evaluations. Women depend on men not so much for financial support as for self-esteem and status. I discuss women's social and emotional dependence on men in the chapter to follow; here I focus on the financial and agentic (self-motivated) dimensions of women's heterosexual partnerships.

The data pertaining to the relationship between money and unsafe sex, described in the section that follows, were collected in phase two of the project, in the clinic.[7] Discourse taken from clinic interview transcripts[8] is presented in tandem with frequencies derived from the questionnaire data (see also Appendix B). Because they are taken from non-random (and, in certain cases, small) samples, the quantitative data are suggestive and informative rather than conclusive[9]; I include them nonetheless as a complement to the rich data contained in the ethnographic narratives that are the preeminent concern of the research and without which the contexts of and reasons for the quantitative findings cannot be fully understood. The similar ways in which the interviewees and questionnaire respondents were recruited and the fact that they were all M&I clients support such cross-referencing.[10]

Condom Use Patterns

Use Rates

Participant condom use rates were quite like those reported elsewhere for similar populations.[11] Eighty-nine of the ninety questionnaire respondents indicated their condom-use patterns on a Likert-type scale. Forty (44.9%) of the eighty-nine used condoms "never" or "rarely"; twenty-nine (32.6%) used them "sometimes" or "often"; twenty (22.5%) used them "very often" or "always." The questionnaire included the standard cross-check inquiry into condom use or non-use during the last sexual encounter, and this provided the basis for grouping the women as users or non-users for the comparisons made below.

Of the ninety questionnaires completed, thirty were pilot and sixty were final-form versions. Among the thirty women who completed the pilot questionnaire, twelve (40%) used condoms during their last sexual encounters; seventeen (56.7%) did not (information was missing for one woman). The final version of the questionnaire asks only sexually active women for information about condom use during their last sexual encounters. I instituted this change to lessen the impact of recall-related

TABLE 2. Condom Use for Sexually-Active Final Questionnaire Respondents and
Clinic Interviewees

	Questionnaire respondents (N=49)	Interviewees (N=25)
Users	11 (22.4%)	7 (28%)
Non-users	38 (77.6%)	18 (72%)

biases on the data collected and to get a clearer picture of the women's
actual and current condom-use patterns. Eleven (18.3%) of the sixty
women were not sexually active.[12] As Table 2 shows, eleven (22.4%) of the
forty-nine respondents who were sexually active said that they used condoms the last time that they had sex; thirty-eight (77.6%) claimed not to
have. Similarly, of the twenty-five clinic interviewees, all of whom were
involved in relationships, seven (28%) said that they had and eighteen
(72%) said that they had not used condoms during their last sexual
encounters.

Women who used condoms during their last sexual encounters ("users") were less likely than those who did not ("non-users") to be involved
in steady conjugal relationships. Furthermore, involved non-users had
been with their partners for much longer than involved users had. Data
from the final questionnaire indicated that significantly more non-users
(58.5%, n = 34) than users (9.1%, n = 11) lived with partners.

According to clinicians, clients report that condom use is harder to
initiate after a relationship has been established than in the early stages
of courtship (see Appendix B1; see also Vander Linden 1993). Client
testimonials about how out of place condoms are in established and
supposedly intact relationships reveal that condoms connote distrust,
disrespect, and disease. Women in long term relationships may be more
dependent on their men for self-esteem and status than women who are
not as involved, and so they may be less willing to confront such connotations. These data regarding condoms' connotations and this relationship
duration hypothesis are important, but before discussing the cultural
and psychosocial dimensions of condom use, which Chapter 7 does, the
association between use rates and financial factors must be scrutinized.

Condom Use and Money

When I began this research I found the popular materialist arguments
compelling. But, contrary to what I originally expected to find, non-use of
condoms was not related to female unemployment. If a relationship between unemployment (financial need) and unsafe sex existed, one would
expect the frequency of non-use to be higher among unemployed women
and lower among the employed. But slightly more non-users than users

had paid jobs. Twenty-five (45.5%) of the fifty-five non-users worked while nine (40.9%) of the twenty-two users did so.[14] This suggestive trend notwithstanding, the employment frequencies are about the same for both users and non-users. Final questionnaire data indicate that users and non-users alike received an average of about one hundred and forty-five dollars each month in financial aid. Further, no significant differences in age, education, number of children, or even age-range of children emerged (however, and as would be expected, non-users were more likely than users to be in the clinic for pregnancy-related care).

Most of the women reported being basically on their own financially. Fifty-four of the ninety questionnaire respondents (60%) were household heads and seventy-five (83.3%) of the ninety women drew resources regularly in their own names. Thirty-eight women (42.2%) brought in paychecks; thirty-six (40%) received only public assistance, one (1.1%) reported both having a job and receiving assistance (here I must note that had we asked directly about food stamps and other non-liquid state or federal assistance, rather than asking about aid in general, the frequency of aid reported probably would have been higher). While incomes varied, data from the final questionnaire[15] suggest that women brought, on average, between three and four hundred dollars into their households monthly from wages, financial assistance checks, and money earned through entrepreneurial activity (e.g., baby-sitting, sewing, doing nails or hair for neighbors) (see Appendix B2).

It must be acknowledged that, despite the guarantee of anonymity, many women may have kept some of their wage and other income secret for fear of being reported to financial assistance or other state authorities. This would lead to a conservative average monthly income figure. Even so, the financial data suggest that women contribute far more to their household budgets than theories focusing on the instrumental patron-client dimension of heterosexual relations imply. And the fact that the women generally see themselves as self-sufficient further suggests that something other than money *per se* may be at the root of unsafe sex.

Betsy, Rose, Nicole

Before discussing in detail the qualitative findings regarding women's financial standings and before presenting their feelings about men and their money, let me introduce a few of the interviewees (brief profiles of all of the clinic interviewees can be found in Appendix A). Betsy, Rose, and Nicole were at different stages of their reproductive careers and differed in age, education, and financial and employment status; they also had rather distinct conjugal partnership styles. Despite these differences, the women shared certain beliefs about themselves and about men — beliefs that many of the other interviewees also held and acted on. Thirty-six-year-old Rose has four children. She is a warm, churchgoing woman. In addition to being one of the oldest women interviewed, Rose also is among the most educated and best paid. Rose has her Associate's degree and works as a receptionist, bringing home $920 each month. She also receives $237 a month in food stamps, and is on what she calls "the budget programs" for gas and electricity. In addition, Rose occasionally works at home as a seamstress.

Rose has been involved with her boyfriend, whom she loves and looks to for companionship, for five years. She and her children live with him in a subsidized apartment. A mechanic, Rose's boyfriend lives up to many of her expectations for men. These pervade the advice that she said she would give to her daughter about them:

I would tell her that he has to have respect for you, to like what you is, to accept you for what you is, [and to be a] hard worker. I feel a hard worker, that's the only way you get anything in life, you know. You have to work towards it, you're not going to get anything laying down on your back. Education is very important to me.

Money "comes in with education and hard work," says Rose, but money should not cause a woman's attraction to a man. Rose's boyfriend helps out by buying shoes for the children now and then, and he pays half the rent and helps with the food bills but, as she points out, he should pay his half because he does live with her. "I really don't use his money, or make him feel like he's my priority as far as finances; I refuse to do that," Rose says, noting that "the kids would help me out." Earlier in the interview she said, "I think that's one thing he likes about me: I don't change my ways when it comes to money, you know, like [if] I know he get paid and I act nice — oh no. If I didn't cook him dinner yesterday, I'm not going to cook [him] dinner tomorrow."

Betsy is ten years younger than Rose. She wears her hair pulled back in a ponytail. Betsy's goals include owning "a nice house, maybe two cars" in the future. At this point in her life, however, she stays with her sister, Bee. Bee does not ask for financial compensation, but Betsy gives Bee the food stamps she receives. This does not amount to much, Betsy says, explaining that "since they [the welfare authorities] found out I was working I only get like $73."

Betsy works part-time for a housekeeping agency and brings home between $350 and $400 a month. "I like to clean," she says, but "I'd rather be a nurse. I'm going to school for a nurse's assistant." Cleaning is "an OK job. I just want something better that pays more, so I don't have to be on welfare any more. I'm very independent."

School is not enjoyable for Betsy because she feels most people there harbor racial prejudices: "If you need something done they can't never find your papers or your records or stuff, things like that; it's always lost for a Black person. They act — they don't speak when you speak to them, like they don't want to be bothered." Still, she plans on persevering in order to better her situation.

Betsy has a boyfriend who helps her out at times but "sometimes he don't, because he tells me that he has other things to do with his money. Buy beer, drink. That's all he does: drink with his friends. Maybe buy like a Walkman. That's the kind of stuff he spends his money on." The two have been together, off and on, for six years. She has given him money at times, and at times, she says, he has squandered that money on other women.

Nicole was twenty years old, pregnant, and fashionably dressed and coifed when we talked. She had worked for four years in a nursing home as an aide. "I really love it," she said, "People hug you all the time. It's not bad. You live and you die and that's where they die at." Despite the fact that "I've always taken care of old people," she dreams of opening her own hairdressing shop.

Nicole, whom I described in my field notes as "bubbly," was fairly social compared to other interviewees. Still, she said, "I don't mix my friends and my man, you know. You can't mix those two things" because of male jealousy and because of the fickleness of female friends. "Why would I promote a problem when it's not necessary?" she asked rhetorically.

At the time of her interview, Nicole's boyfriend was in prison on drug and robbery charges. "We've been together for three [years]," she said, explaining that last year, before he went to jail, "just everything totally changed . . . His friends had just totally just took his mind." After he gets out of prison, she says, the drug-dealing that put him there will be over: "He can get a nice little job somewhere, anywhere, McDonald's, I don't care." As for herself, "I've been working since I was sixteen, you know, and I've always had a social security plan [i.e., a plan for the future, a safety net]."

Condom Use Decisions

Nicole, Betsy, Rose, and the other interviewed women did not feel forced by their partners to do anything that was out of line with their own expectations about appropriate behavior. For example, in response to a question regarding whether or not her partner ever asked her to do anything against her will, Mary shook her head to indicate no and then said, "I'll tell you what he did ask me and beg me and pound it in my head, was to leave drugs alone and learn how to respect myself . . . He never asked me to do anything but be a lady, take care of my son, and keep my respect and honor my mother." These demands demonstrated to her the depth of his love. "He don't ever make a decision or a choice" for me, Mary said. "He just talk to me and I talk to him. . . . He don't give me no decision, 'You should do this,' or 'You shouldn't do that,' or . . . 'I know you want to do it my way.' No."

Regarding sex in particular, Mary never felt pushed by her partner to avoid using condoms. Asked if she ever felt that he might leave her if she did not provide sex the way that he desired it, she said, "Oh no. No. He doesn't want me to disrespect myself. He always says 'Save your soul.' He says, 'Don't ever mess around with nobody that will not honor you, baby, all of you. Save your soul.' You asked me to be frank, right?" Mary continued, explaining that in her view God frowns on certain acts, and pointing out in regard to her partner, "This guy is a man I can talk to."

Like Mary, most of the women did not feel as if they were coerced by their partners into unsafe sex. They did say, however, that *other* men will push for such. Further, as twenty-four-year-old Falasha said, "They lie. They say that they have [condoms] on and. . . . I mean, you want to believe them [but] you can feel it, [and] when they're done—" and she stopped; the outcome was apparent. Linda, also twenty-four, was once tricked into condomless sex: "I said, 'Do you have a condom on?' and he said, 'Yes.' But then, after we started [it turned out that he did not]. . . . I didn't like it and I didn't have sex with him after that." A social-welfare center interviewee told of a time when a male lover who originally agreed to use a condom on his penis "just shoved it in" unsheathed when sex began; this left her quite angry and destroyed the union. Nonetheless, most women claimed to have had condomless sex because they themselves desired or freely agreed to do so.

Indeed, despite the attention paid in the literature to women's need for more male cooperation regarding condom use (Miller et al. 1990, 112; Schneider 1988; Worth 1990), women presented themselves as active players in the sexual arena (cf. Kline et al. 1992). As Table 3 shows, over half (55.6%, n = 30) of the fifty-four questionnaire respondents who provided data about both last condom use and condom use decision making said that the decision to use or not to use condoms is a joint one, made by sexual partners together.[16] With the exception of one woman, a non-user who said that the man decides unilaterally, the remaining twenty-three (42.6%) said that they make the decision for themselves, by themselves.[17] Data collected in phase one was similar (see Appendix B3).

Women who participated in a study of condom use in Philadelphia carried out by Geringer et al. (1993) felt even more independent than the Cleveland women regarding their desires for use or non-use. The Philadelphia study involved 483 Black women. Three hundred and forty

TABLE 3. Self-Reported Decision-Making Style and Condom
Use Among Questionnaire Respondents

	Users (N=23)	Non-users (N=31)
Joint	13 (56.5%)	17 (54.8%)
Self-determined	10 (43.5%)	13 (41.9%)
Male-determined	0	1 (3.2%)

reported ever having used condoms, and these women were asked whose idea condom use generally was. Almost three-fifths (59%) of the women reported making the decision to use condoms by themselves; most of the remaining two-fifths (37%) said that the decision was made jointly. The remaining few said that their partners made the decision.[18] Data concerning who decided about non-use of condoms are not reported. However, Geringer et al. do state that less than 1 percent of the 483 women gave "fear of physical or verbal abuse" as a reason for not using condoms (1993, 81).

Cleveland data suggest that the perceived locus of condom use decision making (whether joint, unilateral, or self-motivated) may not be related to the direction of the use decision choice. As Table 3 shows, of the thirty-one non-using questionnaire respondents for whom decision-making data were available, thirteen (41.9%) reported that they made their decisions by themselves and seventeen (54.8%) said that they made them jointly. In comparison, of the twenty-three users, ten (43.5%) reportedly made their decisions by themselves and thirteen (56.5%) said that they made them jointly. The frequencies are essentially the same.

Adrienne, a mother of three, explained a past unprotected sexual encounter by emphasizing the motivating force of her own sexual drive: "I did it because I wanted to. He didn't make me do it. I wanted to have sex myself at the time." Adrienne was one of the non-users. When asked if she thought that her partner would leave her if she refused to have condomless sex, Adrienne answered, "Nuh-uh. We might have ended up arguing but he's not going to leave, he won't go nowhere." Some non-using women felt that, if they ever did want to use condoms, rather than arguing about it their partners would agree to do so. In the clinic focus group, an apparent non-user said, "He's my mate, and if I ask him and I'm serious about it, he would use a rubber." Another said, "If you sit there for a minute and you tell him that you can't have sex, he'll do it [if he loves you]." But despite — and in many ways because of — the faith that they had in their mates' love for them, most did not desire to use condoms.

Many women said that they had condomless sex because intercourse simply felt better done "skin to skin." In the clinic focus group, a participant said, "I like it better without, 'cause it feels better." Someone responded, "Feel better for who? You or him?" and the woman replied, "Me. What I'm saying is the way I feel about it. It feels like a balloon to me." Others agreed, "A balloon [yes]," "We know it feels better," and "I'd rather have a real skin, flesh against flesh." Chapter 7 returns to the desire for full, barrierless contact and its link to women's faith in their partners' love for them.

Love

What Love Means to Women

Most women felt that they had a large say in the decision not to use condoms, and did not feel forced into condomless sex by financial dependence on men. When asked outright whether it makes a difference if a man has a job, clinic focus group participants responded, "It don't make no difference," "I don't think so," and "What makes a difference is the guy." Another said, "Just [financial] support or nothing ain't got nothing to do with having safe sex with him." Women did mention money when describing their relationships, but they focused more on emotional ties, the personal characteristics of their mates, and the status and self-esteem that being in a relationship brings. Rose, an interviewee who had been with her partner for five years, explained her relationship:

I don't have a mother, [so] I look to him when I'm down. I look to him for companionship. I look to him to lift me up spiritually. [When I] need someone to talk to, I want him to be there to talk to me. Only the true love can understand my feelings, you know. And we agree with each other; we sit down and we talk about it, things like — we shop together, eat together, we go to church together. That's about it, you know. For our sexual lives he's here when I need him.

Love, not money, binds women to men. The support they seek is emotional and social. Betsy says that a partner should be "someone who shares, someone to be there with." She continues, "Love is trust and honesty." June, who works seasonally selling flowers at intersections, noted in her assessment of her partner that he was a "good listener" and a "caring" man who showed his love. When asked for clarification, June provided an example: "If it's like my birthday or something coming 'round, he doesn't necessarily go out and buy me a dozen roses, but the phone rings and he be singing 'Happy Birthday.' " Bernice's partner also was a "romantic type of person," she said "He's the kind of person like a trained [i.e., classy] person, a trained character: bring you roses, sing you verses and stuff like that."

Roberta, who at age thirty-eight was one of the oldest interviewees, said of her partner, "I just like him. I have a lot of fun with him. He has a very nice personality from God." Twenty-four-year-old Linda said that her husband was (and is) "what I really wanted in a relation: someone to spend a lot of time with me, treat me like I was special." Nicole described her boyfriend: "He's smart, for one. He's real, just — he's real sweet, just a sweetheart and everything. . . . He'd never hit me."

Nicole said that men "have to be really responsible. They have to be outgoing. They have to have a personality. They have to have a sense of humor 'cause I would go crazy without a sense of humor. They would have to be educated." She adds, "If he was to drive a truck, he would go out of town and he would come back home and tell me something to broaden my horizons, you know. . . . They got to be able to teach me something." Adrienne also wanted to learn and grow with her partner. She said that she told her daughter,

Get a man who understands you and who will love you as you grow . . . [Find] a guy you can go on a trip with. Your companion is supposed to be like a soul mate . . . Not he go this way, you go that way. You're supposed to go down this path together: sit up and be able to have discussions without arguing, enjoy different programs. A person you enjoy, a person you can communicate with — those are the basics for a good relationship.

Thirty-six-year-old Mary had been off drugs for thirty-three days at the time of her interview. She, too, loved her partner for his teaching — for "doing the man job, making sure I stay out of trouble, talking to me . . . teaching me to the right or wrong, what's good and bad." Bernice cast her partner as a bit of a teacher as well; she said that he "taught me a lot about love that I didn't know." I asked, "You mean the physical act of love?" and she said, "Everything, just pure in general."

While the interviewed women had various definitions of love, most were basically similar. Mary said, "Love means to me someone to talk to, to hold, to cherish, to understand me, to honor me, to be honest to me." She loves her partner because "he's a hell of a man. 'Cause he stuck by me [when I was on drugs] and I kept telling him that I was no good for him and he said, 'No baby, you all right, you'll learn and I'm here to help you because I love you.' "

Shelly, who was twenty-three and who, six months prior to the interview, had been in prison for drug and robbery charges, also valued her partner's caring attitude, "His best qualities really is [his asking if] I'm all right. He's worrying about me — physically, mentally, romantically; he's worrying if I'm OK." Like Shelly and Mary, most women definitely saw emotional supportiveness as an attractive feature in men.

Love, said thirty-six-year-old Dee, who had been with her partner for nineteen years, means "two people just sharing, two people so together that they share one soul basically, that everything — they work things out. . . . Love's just something between two people, I guess those two only really know." Dee said, "If I ever need something, like if something hurt me, he can tell. He can tell that something is bothering me, and he can really dig down to the point and get it out of me and fix it for me."

Most of the interviewees with children mentioned that they loved how their partners acted toward their children. Linda, who at twenty-four had two children and a full-time job as a secretary, said of her husband, "He's a good father to our children. He takes a lot of time with them as well as me." Later, she explained,

I really didn't have my father when I was growing up and I promised myself that if and when I got married I would always want my husband to be a good father. And he spends time with them, and he talks with my children; he reads books to them, he just spends a lot of time for them. And also I don't have to do all the work: when they were younger he made bottles — just as many bottles as I did. He changed them just as many times as I did, you know. Basically, he works a different shift: I work eight to four-thirty, he works three to eleven. So I get their clothes ready and he basically gets them dressed and takes them to the babysitter. So I don't have to worry about that. He does a lot for them. He shares the responsibility.

Donna, a thirty-four-year-old mother of six, said of her new boyfriend, "He's real gentle. He's bright. He likes my kids." Bernice, who at twenty-four had one daughter, said of her beau: "He's good with kids." She liked the way that her partner managed his own home life; he treated his own children as well as he treated her little girl. She said, "He is a calm person. He likes to be at home, satisfy his children, take time out with them." Later, she said, "He's like a family man."

Twenty-one-year-old Sarah, who dreamed of being a nurse, talked about love and her partner:

He's always supporting me with whatever choice I choose. I do the same for him, I'm always there for him. [If we] need advice, [we] sit down and talk about things. . . . It's just like being in heaven, you know. It's nice, it's wonderful! It's just a nice feeling, waking up knowing that, 'Wow, I got a guy who really cares for me.' I can do something with a guy instead of walking around being with girls.

Sarah's last statement indicates that being "with a guy" brings status in a way that "being with girls" does not.

Like the interviewees, focus group participants looked for men who treated them well. "It would have to do with the way he treats you," one clinic woman said, adding "a lot of times the woman can be so turned on by the way he treats her that . . . it feel good when he touch." So relationships, and the sexual intimacy they entail, can follow from emotional and personality factors rather than financial ones. As another participant said, "You know, before I really got into sex, [I saw that] he got good values and morals that I like in him as a man." Another woman echoed this opinion; she said, "I appreciate a man for his values." Someone immediately added, "Where you all share the overall outlook on life."

Love and Stupidity

Some of the women pointed out that love can lead to foolish thoughts and actions. Marvelle, who was twenty-one and pregnant with her first child, said that when you are in love, "you do just about anything for them. You want to do a whole bunch of garbage that you really shouldn't, because you love him." Talk in the clinic focus group led to similar conclusions. For example, one woman said, "A woman can love a man so much that she just don't worry about [AIDS]." Another said, "If you love him and you're all infatuated with him, you probably would say 'OK, come on back here' [after your partner had an affair] because you're in love — you're stupid. You're stupid, you're infatuated."

Many women mentioned friends in such situations. Interviewee Linda's friend Ronnie, for example, had hooked herself up with a man who is

not a good husband; he's really bad. [Interviewer: "What makes him not a good husband?"] He cheats on her, doesn't spend any time with her, doesn't help with the child they have, doesn't buy anything for the child, or spend time with the child. [They still live together but] I don't understand why. I think she thinks she loves him. To me personally, how can you love somebody that does that to you?

The element of unfaithfulness plays a large part in many of the interviewees' stories about friends who both do "garbage" and put up with it because of love — a point that I shall return to in the next chapter as I discuss the impact of a mental process called the "optimistic bias" on condom use rates.

Another interviewee, Betsy, had her own "garbage" story to tell: she said that she stays with a mentally and physically abusive partner even though he gives her no money and even though she knows that she would be welcome to stay with her relatives, because she loves him. Betsy was even "buying him things like clothes, anything he wanted he got it. [Interviewer: "Why was that?"] Because I love him." She finally stopped "because I seen that he didn't want to do anything for himself."

Money

Thirty two (72.7%) of the forty-four questionnaire respondents who provided explicit income data said that they received some financial help from men. Twelve (27.3%), however, did not. Proportionally more non-users than users received money, but users who did receive cash got, on average, surprisingly more from men than non-users did (for exact figures and regarding frequencies reflecting the entire sample of ninety, see Appendix B2).

Although almost three in four women received at least some money from men, more than one in four did not. Very few interviewees pointed to the attractiveness of men's money when talking about their partners' best qualities. Men's money was seen by users and non-users alike as either a personal perk—perhaps used as a tool for showing love (more of which below)—or as a household contribution (for child-related expenses or rent) that is rightfully due when a man and woman live or have children together. But in either case it was not to be counted on.

Sarah talked about important male traits without mentioning money, so I asked about it directly; she said, "No, it ain't never been a money thing. When I first met him he ain't had nothing, you know. He didn't have a job—he was going to school but he didn't have a job, so it never worked that way." Dee responded to a similar probe with a perplexed shake of the head and then asked me "What do I need him for? I'm going to have to go home and think about this. I don't know. He doesn't pay bills. I need him for sex!" Earlier, she'd explained, "I have a boyfriend [but] I don't depend on him as far as financial-wise because he's into splurging." Other interviewees also told of partners more interested in buying things for themselves than for the women or their children.

If interviewees did bring up men's money as an attraction, it was usually in the context of an explanation of the good things that the willingness and ability to work say about a man (or in the context of talk about gifts or dinner dates, which I shall return to later). Still, the women felt that jobs are not always easy to come by, and so they did not interpret unemployment itself as a bad sign regarding a man's character. "Take a man as whatever they are, not for what they got. Take them for what they are and then work from there," advised Bernice. "Work on it and eventually he'll get [a job]. You just don't kick him to the curb," said Mary.

Weighing carefully the question of whether or not she could see herself falling in love with a jobless man, Linda said, "It depends on if they were in school or not."

If they're in school trying to do something [yes, I can see it]. But somebody who just didn't have a job and who wasn't trying to find a job, then no. But if they didn't have a job for the time being, you know, [if] they're in between jobs [then yes]. [But] if they're a certain kind of people. . . . If they just didn't have a job at all—then no, I wouldn't be interested in them. They're not trying, they're not doing anything for themselves so, you know, how could they do something for me, I mean motivate me. I want someone who's gonna motivate me and be there for me. Having no job, that would make me lose a little respect for him because he's not trying. And I don't need nobody pulling me down. [Interviewer: "You mean bringing you down financially?"] Emotionally too. If they don't have a job they're always depending on you. That's kind of emotional for you. You don't want anybody that's always pulling you down.

Shelly, who was trying to "make a way" and to "better" herself now that she was out of prison, said that it was important that her partner worked and brought in money, because "he's a good role model for me."

If a man who did not go to school just could not find work, he could keep house. Adrienne, whom I described in my notes as "motherly," said, "If he didn't have a job [but] I come home to a clean house and some food like he would want to come home to, that would be OK. See, I understand the big city world." Adrienne recognized that modern urban life demands flexibility.

Men should work if they can, but most women talked about sharing the burden of providing for a family. Penny said, "I think it should be fifty-fifty, you know, 'cause I wouldn't want a man to have all that pressure." "The man and the woman ought to pull together," Donna declared. Roberta stated, "It takes two incomes to run a household." "[One] income alone wouldn't do it," said Linda. Both she and her husband worked full-time. She explained that there's "more money, of course, if I always work," seconds after proclaiming, "I get a satisfaction from it. I enjoy working and I wouldn't want to be a housewife 'cause it's boring, you know."

Mary saw purposeful female unemployment negatively, as a sign of a woman's selfishness and of her flawed understanding of what a good relationship should entail:

You could have a man be good to you all your life [financially] and then you have your own [money] and you be selfish, and one day that man can get his arm cut off on the job, get run over, get paralyzed, and you think that you not supposed to be able to take care of him like he took care of you? No, I think that it should be equal. Equal. My man help me, I help my man. We're both supposed to be in there together. He isn't supposed to give me everything he got and then I keep all mine. No, 'cause see one day anything can happen, you know; it's not going [to be easy] all the time. We should share with each other. I don't want to be with no one I can't share and be comfortable with.

Another interviewee, Dee, explained further that sharing expenses is important because it reduces the distance between people: "Because that way you don't have to say 'This is totally mine and this is totally yours.' [Instead, you can say] 'This is ours together, we both put in together.'" As mentioned, Dee saw love as "two people so together that they share one soul."

Michelle also felt that sharing the burden of bread-winning equally was best: "It's way too hard on one person." Moreover, Michelle felt that she would not like being kept by a man. "I just don't like that. As long as I'm healthy and able to work I will work." Nicole, whose boyfriend was in jail, said just about the same thing, "I don't want to be like that, no . . . I want to have my career and I want to do what I want to do." Basically, so did every other interviewee.

All the interviewees had plans for their futures that included financial independence and, in some cases, home ownership. Twenty (80%) of the twenty-five women saw themselves as already financially independent. "You don't need a man to take care of you. You get out here and do it for yourself," said Dee, later adding, "I guess my parents raised us to be self-dependent and that's all I've ever known: 'Get out there and get what you want for yourself.' " Earlier she had noted, "What the man give you, that be your pleasure money."

Ruth, a mother of one who just had major surgery and whose husband was too busy drinking to worry about his responsibilities (or her well-being), declared, "When I need stuff I just buy it out of my own money." So does Clarissa, who, twenty-eight and expecting her fourth child, gets food stamps and welfare. She says:

I'm the whole family, yeah. [My husband] keeps calling me the man of the house. I feel like I'm doing a good job. I was telling my kids the other day, I said, 'Whenever you need something,' — they don't have the most expensive clothes, but when I really need something, like paper, books, [or] shoes, I get it.

Marvelle echoed this sentiment: "The welfare is [minimal]," she said, "but I do know how to budget money. I don't actually depend on [my partner]."

The majority of the women had strategies for financial survival. Dee said, "I go to garage sales or yard sales." Clarissa explained, "I keep food stamps. When I get them, I go to the grocery store, get something. But the prices go down after a certain time of the month so I give my sister $200 or $100 to hold for me, and then by the time end of the month comes, like I say, I got food."

Adrienne budgeted well too. She said, "I'm a pretty good shopper," later adding, "We have to set limits on how we budget our lifestyle. We pretty much have one night out a week. It's our family night. Usually we go to Burger King." Adrienne did not receive help from her boyfriend or from anyone else: "I just do like I do on my own. I pretty much manage it." She did receive some state aid; of this, she said, "It's not much, but I do with what I have, and I play bingo and I play a little lottery sometime" in an effort to extend the cash.

Most of the women pointed out that at times making ends meet could be difficult. Penny was in worse financial shape than most of the interviewees: she had just left her husband of seven years because his crack-cocaine habit made him intolerable and dangerous. When asked about finances, she confided, "Sometimes at night, especially after a day like today, I cry. I don't cry just for things like that [Penny's three-year-old had just upset Ms. Dayse's desk], but I cry when I get real upset, like 'Why should I have to do it on my own?' " But like the others, Penny enjoyed the feeling of self-sufficiency that smart budgeting and being able to provide for oneself and one's children brings. "It makes me feel good," she said.

"It's such a good thing you can't even describe how good it feels," said Nicole. "I feel good because I've been doing it for so long. Like feeding my children, I learned to do those things," said Adrienne, adding, "I've always worked, but I got more independent after he got incarcerated, 'cause there was nobody else."

Donna, who sometimes received financial help from her partner, also received it from her relatives. "One day," she said, when she was visiting her mother,

I was like, "I got to get some jackets for my kids," and I says, "I don't think [the baby] has a jacket". . . . So that evening, my ma came over and she brought forty dollars. She said, "Hey, you could give the baby a jacket." She always—she's there, you know.

Donna continued, saying,

My grandmother, she tries to be a little too helpful. . . . When I go to see my grandma I can't have—I can't go and say, "Oh man, I got to go buy my kids some tennis shoes, [I don't know] where to get the money from," 'cause she'll just want to—she'll give you the money. And I don't like for her to feel she has to always do for me.

Donna had gone through some very hard times earlier. She said of her mother and other relatives, "They had to take the load on their backs. That made me feel kind of sad . . . So now it feels good to be able to pay my bills, and . . . take care of my kids the way they are supposed to be taken care of." Although this chapter focuses on women's relationship to men, I have inserted these stories of Donna's female kin to show that women do receive help from relatives as well as from partners and, moreover, to demonstrate that some of the same issues that affect women's feelings about being granted money by men affect their feelings about financial favors done for them by women. Maintaining a sense of independence seems imperative.

"Being independent, it's just like an inside victory, you know," said Roberta, who further explained:

I feel like I am my own woman. When you're independent, you stand on your own two feet. When I [find] a man that takes that away from me — you know, do so much for you till you feel dependent on him — I don't know if I would let anybody do that because I like being independent. I feel strong. I don't feel like I'm better than no one else but I just feel strong within myself.

Roberta did think about the money that her partner brought into her household and she did try to change her sexual behavior for him at one point:

He likes to have sex every day. [I felt like if I agreed and] did it like that [every day] that he would stay. And I know that if he stayed that his money would stay. [But] he started getting on my nerves [and so] by November he was out.

So Roberta would get money from her partner, but she did not rely on it, and when the cost of its extraction disagreed with her, she kicked him out. She did not compromise herself for money.

Finding a Man

For Roberta, as for Penny[18] — that is, for two in twenty-five women — trading (or not trading) sex for money was a pragmatic matter. For others, it was a moral issue. A clinic focus-group participant saw the male partner as the immoral one, particularly if he required condomlessness as part of the bargain: "What kind of mate would use a condom like that?" A fellow participant said, "A [man] like that is an immature person who can't see." But most participants focused on the woman's moral position. As twenty-four-year-old Bernice, a mother of one, explained in relation to the thought of trading sex, with or without a condom, for money,

I don't think it's right, I think that's just using people. My girlfriend's mother used to try to set me up with this older man 'cause he had money but I couldn't do it. If I didn't have [money] then I didn't have it, but I'm not going to bed or doing nothing with no man just to make no money.

Women's stories about how they met their partners revealed little evidence of overt money-driven manipulation. For instance, Adrienne met her partner at a restaurant:

[He] said, "Young lady how are you today?" and I said "Fine." He said, "Is your husband married?" and I said, "I don't know that." I said, "Are you and your wife married?" and he said, "My wife's divorced." He said, "Can I give you a phone call?" and I said, "Yeah."

Ruth met her partner when she was in another relationship. She explained,

[I] talked to him on the phone for six months before [going out with] him, and we talked about—I was going—I was in a relationship and I would talk to him. He was more of a person that would listen.

Like Ruth, a number of other women reported meeting their current partners while still with or just separated from previous ones. Rather than women appearing predatory, men seemed to be the ones on the lookout for partners. They often entered women's lives by moving in to fill other men's freshly emptied (or nearly emptied) shoes—sometimes slowly, sometimes with haste. Roberta said, "I had just lost my husband . . . we just started being together . . . He would know that I'm feeling bad or something and he would sing me something real silly . . . to bring me out of my depression." Nicole met her present boyfriend when she was getting ready to go to the prom with her previous boyfriend (note that she and not the old boyfriend funded the outing):

I was putting gas in my rental car and . . . he was like, "Hi. Your hair looks good." And I was like, "Yeah." He was just getting gas . . . Like for a year me and my boyfriend were—I was still going with my other boyfriend then. [So the present one and I] would just talk on the phone, you know, and then we would go like to the show every [so often] and then we [got together] . . . Just everything totally changed. It was like we had a different mentality, and it was just—[we were] just into each other.

Talking on the phone prior to dating, as both Ruth and Nicole did, was common. Michelle met her beau at a party "just walking around, talking to people, and somebody introduced us. I thought he was cute. We exchanged phone numbers and we talked on the phone for a couple weeks and [then] went out on a couple of dates." Sex started three months after that.

Linda, who was married, met her partner on a blind date. "My friends had set us up," she said. "We went out to the restaurant Friday evening and we hit it off from there and he was just so nice." They spent the whole night socializing: they ate and made merry with two other couples and "then after that, it was like six of us, we all went out to breakfast." Meeting through friends or relatives was common. But, like Nicole above, some women met their partners on their own. Donna met her partner grocery shopping:

I was in the grocery store and he was buying meat, and he asked me what was a rump roast. He was serious! He didn't know. Goofy. I told him once, "You're so goofy." [And] I told him—I was teasing him; I said, "You weren't trying to flirt with me or anything: you wanted to know about that piece of meat!"

Still, although Donna met her partner on her own, it turned out that "he takes bible studies at this church where my mama teaches. He goes to church with my mother." In many cases, social links were known to exist prior to a conjugal connection.

Participants did say that some women sought men out for money or acquiesced to their men's demands for condomless sex because they did not want to lose the resources that their men provided them with. Clinic focus group participants said such behavior was related to "lifestyle." Asked what that meant, one participant said that the woman who did a man's bidding for financial gain was "a drug user, number one, and a prostitute, number two." Another woman shook her head and said, "No morals," and someone else added, "A woman that really don't care." One participant said,

If she can get that money, living that lifestyle, and that man tells her he ain't gonna give it — cause she won't get the money if he gotta use a rubber — he won't use that rubber, and he's gonna get sex without that rubber and she's gonna get her money.

Participants held exchanging unsafe sex for money to be a practice confined to a different, and a lesser, class of women. Further, interviewees generally felt gold-digging to be a foolish and contemptible idea. Shelly said, "Those thoughts have come to my mind, but I never changed my way because I find that if I change my way he'd be leaving anyway." Regarding the question of sex for financial gain, Mary said, "Oh no, I can't do anything like that. I will help somebody cleaning house or help somebody watch their kids [instead]."

While money is indeed appreciated, most women felt that money is no panacea. As Mary said, "You can have all the money in the world and be very, very sad and unhappy." Linda's words echoed this sentiment: "It takes more than to just bring home some money. I mean, you have to spend time with your spouse and communicate. I think that's the major thing." Dee advised me, protectively, "Don't get a man just for money-wise."

Men's Money: Necessity or Luxury?

The interviewees who received money from their partners said that they did not need this money and they did not manipulate their men to get it, but they also did not refuse it. Even Dee said, "I'm no fool — I'm not going to turn it down." Vicki said almost the exact same thing: "I just take it anyway. I don't turn nothing down. If he's gonna give me something then I have it." Twenty-one-year-old Sarah, who made about $200 a month doing hair for girlfriends, got about $75 every two weeks from her boyfriend. But, she explained, "I don't expect it. It really don't matter, you know. If he gives it to me, he gives it to me, and if he don't, he don't." In that case, she said, "I just wait and something happens, or I do some-body's hair and there's $45." Sarah spelled things out:

You see, I'm my own woman. I don't [mind] him helping me out or taking care of me, [but] when you depend on people that slows you down. If you need some-thing done — like say if I had my own place and I'm dependent on him to give me this $70, $80 to pay a phone bill or a gas or a light bill, and then he can't give it to me, that's making me mess up, slowing my pace. . . . [I'd rather] pay it then don't have to worry about it none. So I don't depend on him too much, you know.[19]

Like Sarah, Donna does hair for a fee: "I put braids in people's hair; [it's] something I can do at home . . . If I do braids, I'll do — I'll start like about 8:30 in the morning, and I'll get finished at about 8:00 at night. Maybe two, three days a week. [People pay] about $85 to $100." Her partner gives her money now and then, "or he'll bring fried chicken or Chinese food or something like that." Further, as he works downtown, he sometimes stops in at the utility companies and "pays my cable bills for me and pays my telephone bills." But she does not depend on him. "He don't understand why I won't let him help a little more than what he does," she says. "I told him, 'I'm just used to being independent.' And I don't need him to give [to] me. I need him for friendship and companionship."

One of the main reasons for wanting to be "independent" is uncer-tainty: men employed or devoted today may be neither employed nor devoted tomorrow. I already mentioned Mary's concern over accidents ("that man can get his arm cut off on the job"). As Shelly said of male provisioning, "There's gonna be a time when he ain't gonna be able to do that, you know." Beside getting hurt or growing old, men can (and do) leave. Michelle observed, "There may not be a significant other so there-fore you might have to be the one to take care of yourself."

The acknowledged uncertainty of inner-city life and of love (and so of men's caretaking efforts) made the ability to provide for one's own house-hold crucial, and attaining the sense of achievement (Roberta's "inside victory") that self-sufficiency brought was important to the women. So was avoiding the self-loathing that financial dependence can engender. Se-rious, soft-spoken, self-sufficient Bernice describes the loss of self-esteem that dependence can bring and that she, like all of the other women, would rather avoid. She also comments on the fickleness of men:

I would be disgusted with myself. I just wouldn't feel good 'cause I made myself bound and my child bound. [I'd] feel like I'd be going backwards instead of forwards. I want to be a strong person and not so much dependent on other people to help me out. I feel good when somebody got their hand out asking me for something, that feels good, you know, that somebody can count on me. It's not wrong or anything [to count on somebody], but sometime in your life you just got to stop and do something for your own self. I have never counted on my baby's father, you know, never count on him. He did try to do his part and I appreciate that, but I never counted on him. [If I would have waited] on him to bring Pampers or milk, my baby would fall asleep soaking [and hungry]. You can't wait like that—you got things to do, people to take care of.

Despite their own poverty, some of the women even managed to help take care of people less fortunate than themselves. Adrienne, for example, helped cook meals for the homeless at her church.

As Kline et al. point out in a 1992 paper that is an exception to the rule, scholars investigating unsafe sex have generally represented Black women as financially and structurally dependent on men when this may not be the common case. Like the women in the Kline et al. study, the Cleveland interviewees present themselves as able and willing to take care of themselves. Indeed, they need to be. As mentioned, unemployment, incarceration, and homicide rates make "good" male partners hard to come by in the inner city. This demographic (and, ultimately, epidemiological) fact plus the women's testimony undermine simple materialist models of risky sex and support the argument that emotional and social dependence play a much greater role in encouraging AIDS-risk denial.

Men's Non-Cash Contributions

Estimated Rates

Women explained that they did not actually depend on men's money, making specific reference to their own self-esteem as well as to the high risks that relying on male aid would involve. But even those women dead-set against the idea that they depended on their men financially talked freely of male gifts in kind (generally, clothing and dinners out). This suggests that male gifts have a special psychocultural significance. It also suggests that focusing on dollar amounts when trying to gauge women's reliance on men blinds researchers to many kinds of valued contributions.

To determine the possible importance of non-financial or indirect aid for the women and to ascertain its range, the women were asked to estimate, on ten Likert-type scales, how often their partners gave them ten specified types of resources or aid (regarding cash contribution data, see Appendix B2). Women were asked how often they received food, clothing, intravenous or other drugs, small appliances, entertainment, help with repairs, help with the children or housework, or other kinds of presents or aid from their partners. They were also asked whether they received help with their bills. The possible answers provided in the five-part Likert-type scale for each question ranged from "never" to "very often," with "rarely," "sometimes," and "often" in between. Data were available from seventy-five women: twenty-two users and fifty-three non-users of condoms.

The answer patterns for condom users and non-users were skewed slightly in opposite directions, although they did not follow perfect curves. Non-users most frequently said that they received offerings or favors from their partners "very often" (27.4%, N = 379 answers given), users most frequently said that they "never" received these (37.7%, N = 154 answers given). Users most frequently reported receiving entertainment. Clothing and small household goods are the next most commonly mentioned items. For non-users, the top gift was food, followed by clothing and entertainment (see Appendix B4).

Interview discourse revealed that women give men gifts and provide them with goods and favors too. Betsy's habit of "buying [her partner] things like clothes, anything he wanted" was already mentioned. Other women did the same. Bernice said of her beau, "I helped him. He moved in with me and my boarder." Adrienne said, "I was spending my money, taking him out to dinner, buy new clothes, long johns, PJs, you name it. I got his little girl some dresses." Earlier, she said that gift exchange was important for a relationship: "He buys it first and she buy him a gift you know. It should be even." But this did not prove to be so in her relationship, as her partner rarely reciprocated and he took advantage of her good will. "I was helpful and that was wrong," Adrienne said in hindsight.

It may be that gifts given to men by women equal or outweigh the gifts that men give to women. However, the importance of discerning this was not anticipated when the study was planned as materialist models were not originally under scrutiny and because of this, and because men did not use the M&I clinics and so were not recruited for the study, men's reports of gifts received were not collected. Data from men should be gathered in the future.[20]

Presents and Power

Nice as they may be, in-kind items or favors bestowed are not liquid like cash. While women can allocate cash as they see fit, gifts in kind or of labor position women as wards, with little liberty to manage their own affairs or to make decisions regarding spending priorities. And, as with most charity cases, the recipients—the women—often have little say about important details such as the style of dress received, or the kind of food that partners bring them to cook, or when the year-old hole in the door will get fixed. This plus the lack of liquidity may lessen the practical value of male offerings to women, and such offerings may be experienced as indexing controlling or oppressive relations. In light of this, the fact that on average condom-users received more from men in cash (see Appendix B2) and less in kind than non-users received takes on an unforeseen importance.

Bernice, whom we met above, described the power plays that accompany accepting gifts of any kind from men: "They think they have the upper hand or something." They will "get all worked up and stuff, 'Well, I did this for you,' and stuff like that, trying to make theyself look big." Rose felt the same way: "He would be domineering and then, see, I don't like that." But women especially disliked having to ask for particular gift items because this seemed to magnify men's power more. Rachel, a mother of two who had just entered a drug addiction recovery program, explained her feelings with examples:

[You feel] "Oh I need these shoes," and then you have to explain why you gotta have this other pair of shoes and they know you got other shoes in the closet. . . . I didn't like to have to go and explain to him why I wanted to go get this or that. To go through with him [demanding], "What's wrong with this dress here?" When you got your own money you're in control.

Presents and Love

Despite the fact that in certain circumstances men's gifts can be experienced as controlling or as signs of men's "domineering," men's gifts can also hold an abundance of positive emotional value for women: they can be taken as welcome signals of love and good intentions. A man who gives his wife or girlfriend gifts, services, or money lives up to — or at least begins to live up to and implies that he intends to live up to — the cultural ideal of the male partner as a breadwinner or a provider and as a woman's protector. Their extraconjugal sex habits notwithstanding, men can demonstrate through benefaction that they care. This may be one reason for women's ostentatious display of certain kinds of male gifts to them, such as finger rings.[21]

For Mary, who often got her meals at soup kitchens and her clothes from donation bins, gifts like shoes for bare feet were more precious than rings. As we talked about her relationship, I asked her to explain what she meant by "love" and by "doing the man job," a phrase she used to describe one of her partner's most attractive traits. Mary explained that he protected or guided and provided for her, and she gave examples: "If I need some shoes or my son needs some shoes, or I need to go to the doctor or I need some food, and to keep me out of trouble and to be there for me . . . Talking to me, bringing things to me."

To double-check Mary's meaning, I suggested that there were two sides to her relationship, an emotional side and a practical side. But Mary cut me off when I suggested that his giving and her receiving shoes was pragmatic, saying, "No, that's love. When your man love you and he see you need some shoes he get it for you if he — how could he love you and let you go and neglect yourself? That's not love. That's just using you for your body, for sex." Adrienne succinctly summed up what Mary and the other women felt: "If a man don't give you no money, he don't care nothing about you."

Presents are taken to symbolize love. They are not the only way that a partner can demonstrate love and affection. But they seem to be an important way, especially for women who do not use condoms. In the final questionnaire, women in relationships were asked how their partners showed them love. Most women (35.9%, N = 39) said that their partners did this by meeting their emotional needs. Meeting material needs ran a close second (30.8%). Proportionally more non-users that condom users said that their partners showed love in the latter fashion (see Appendix B5).

Women who do not use condoms might focus more on material indexes of love than users do because more of their partners apparently tend to use gifts and money to demonstrate love. But other factors, such as expectations, might also explain the different rates of reported gift-giving for users and non-users. Many women need to see and to have others see their partners as fulfilling the faithful provider role — as doing what non-user Mary called "the man job." These needs might lead such women to request or require (whether overtly or covertly) more gifts from their men. Or these needs might, in certain contexts, lead some women — especially those who have few other sources for status and self-esteem — to exaggerate or pay more attention to male gifts of cash or kind. Doing so inadvertently lends support to one-dimensional instrumental explanations of unsafe sexual behavior that cast women as totally materially dependent while ignoring both the expressive dimension of reciprocity and the income women have independent of men.

Exaggerations of or selective attention to gifts also helps women maintain their denial of AIDS risk, which characteristically requires constant reinforcement ("You see, he *does* love me") and which entails unsafe sex (I explain these claims in Chapter 7). Moreover, when men give presents wives and girlfriends may, in turn, demonstrate that they trust in their partners' interest in their welfare by reciprocating for that love with condomless sex.

There is, as I have shown, more to romance than finance: condomless sex is not directly purchased. Women may capitulate more readily to partners' demands for unsafe sex when partners give them resources because such giving is seen to entail love and the fulfillment of duty. Male provisioning is seen to imply caring and respect—qualities unexpected from adulterous men. Women reckon that partners who look like they intend to provide support do love them and do not intend to have sex with outside partners. The receipt of male offerings and favors can lead to unsafe sex while simultaneously reinforcing the same denial of AIDS risk that women actively use unsafe sex to bolster.

Discussion

A man's love for his partner is indexed in the offerings he makes to her and the favors that he grants her (regarding the expressive value of reciprocity and gift-giving, see Bailey 1971; Mauss 1967; Sobo 1993b). The social desirability of male contributions and women's selective memories relative to this desirability may lead, in certain contexts, to exaggerated claims of male gift-giving—claims that hide the low value and infrequency of men's contributions to their households and so seem to support a materialist model of romantic involvement (for another example of the impact of social desirability on women's reports of male financial input, see Rubin 1976).

Despite the cultural importance of male provisioning, the findings presented suggest that inner-city women generally consider themselves self-sufficient and independent from men financially. They have a firm sense of agency and they see themselves as active participants in sexual decisions. Love and the trust that it involves, rather than money, is the immediate root of unsafe sex.

One last datum needs to be mentioned in relation to women's self-concept: it seems that self-identifying as African American rather than as Black may be linked with the propensity to use condoms. This finding was made accidentally. While questionnaire respondents only had the option of checking off that they were "Black," "white," or "other; please explain," which were the options preferred by M&I staff members on the basis of their experience with a wide cross-section of clients, clinic interviewees were asked what race or ethnic group that they would say they belonged to. The interviewees could self-identify in any way they wanted. Twelve (48%) of the twenty-five clinic interviewees self-identified as African American and ten (40%) self-identified as Black. But of the seven condom users in the sample, five (71.4%) self-identified as African American. By examining the data from another angle, we see that, while seven women in the whole clinic interviewee sample (28%) used condoms, five (41.7%) of the twelve self-identified African American women did so. A relationship between pro-active ethnic identity politics and condom use may exist.[22]

My findings suggest that the implied tie between unsafe sex and money is only loosely bound; moreover, it is mediated by social and psycho-cultural factors. While the potential for financial gain through heterosexual relations does exist and may be fantasized about just as women can dream about true love and high prestige, in reality—as reflected in the numbers of participants working or bringing in government aid—and despite the obstacles of sexism, poverty, and racism, many inner-city women can and do actively seek support by themselves, in their own names. Generally, however, women cannot gain status and emotional fulfillment on their own. That tends to require a heterosexual relationship with a man, as the next chapter shows.

*   *   *

Much of the material in this chapter was adapted from "Finance, Romance, Social Support, and Condom Use Among Impoverished Inner-City Women," *Human Organization* 54 (2) (1995): 115–128.

Notes

1. Women's risk for HIV infection rises with male incarceration rates, because homosexual relations are common among men in prison.

2. A segment of sexuality research investigates knowledge, attitudes, and beliefs as correlates of sexual practices (e.g., House et al. 1990; Timberlake and Carpenter 1991; Weinberg and Williams 1988). Topics are generally investigated with survey research methods, which measures such things as levels of agreement with given statements or self-reported frequencies of behaviors. As this research is quantitative, little effort is made to illuminate the meanings behind the numbers presented.

3. Still, as psychological and cultural factors are indeed generally mentioned, few (if any) scholars can be said to promote super-simplistic materialist models in which cultural and psychological elements have no play at all.

4. Even with high levels of self-efficacy, other risks can intervene. As so many have noted, the risk of HIV infection is but one of many that impoverished inner-city women face regularly. Moreover, HIV's future consequences are not immediately felt as hunger and coldness are. These reasons have been used widely to explain why women rarely take sexual AIDS-risk reduction steps (Fullilove et al. 1990; Mays and Cochran 1988; Tunstall et al. 1991; Worth 1989; see also Ward 1993b).

5. Multiple partnering is correlated with a tendency to forgo condoms (Catania et al. 1992). A whole behavioral constellation traceable to life chances and childhood experience might be behind this: writing about African-Caribbean men in

Barbados, Handwerker (1993) discusses the link between men's perceived disempowerment, perceptions of childhood abuse, male desires to abuse women, and unsafe sex elected by men. Similar patterns may exist in the United States (regarding African American men's heightened need to dominate women, see Anderson 1990, 118–120; Worth 1990).

6. Blacks were underrepresented (by about half) in Blumstein and Schwartz (1983, as cited in Turner et al. 1989, 110–11), education levels were higher than average for our participants and, because of sampling methods, the study is not generalizable. But it is the only study to my knowledge that explores extraconjugal affairs among unmarried, cohabiting couples as well as married ones. As the figures do not include non-cohabiting couples, of which there are many in poor, urban communities, I also cited Bower (1991), whose figures apply to both white and African American men. I should note that a "substantial" number of heterosexually coupled men have bisexual affairs (Muir 1991, 91; Turner et al. 1989, 152). Covert bisexuality is probably more common among Black than white men because of the ways that Black identity is constructed (Dalton 1989; Mays and Cochran 1990; Mays 1989).

7. I present these findings now (rather than waiting until after I have presented the first-phase data) in order to establish directly the limitations of a purely materialist framework.

8. Most of the interview material included in this paper is transcribed verbatim from audio tapes, but repetitions and some of the more non-grammatical linguistic twists are excluded for ease in reading where doing so does not alter meanings. Pseudonyms rather than real names are given.

9. The quantitative data are presented as raw numbers, or in tandem with simple frequencies to aid in comparisons. No findings from statistical tests are provided here because that would be uninformative and even misleading.

10. While some of the women who completed the questionnaire were not in relationships, all interviewees were; interview data are used accordingly to avoid generating moot hypotheses.

11. Comparing reported condom use rates is a treacherous undertaking, as different studies use different methods to elicit this information and women's feelings about the studies and so their honesty will vary. But it seems that an average of about 20 to 25 percent of poor urban minority women claim always to use condoms. The lower end of the range is seen in Catania et al. (1993), who report that 14 percent use condoms always, 26 percent use them sometimes, and 60 percent never use them; the higher end is seen in Geringer et al. (1993), who describe a "trichotomy" in which approximately one-third of the sample used condoms consistently, one-third used them sometimes, and one-third never used them.

12. This figure might have actually been higher: thirteen women (21.7%) claimed not to be sexually active when asked directly elsewhere in the questionnaire. The figure given, eleven, was derived from a portion of the questionnaire dealing with condom-use decisions. Only sexually active women were asked to provide answers for that section, because otherwise the possibility of recall-related errors would have been higher and also because celibate women are at a much lower risk for AIDS. Forty-nine respondents provided answers for that section.

13. Both employment and use data were available for seventy-seven questionnaire respondents. Beside those who worked, thirty non-users (54.5%, N = 55) and thirteen users (59.1%, N = 22) did not.

14. Forty-four sexually active women provided explicit financial information on the final questionnaire, which was revised with the need for such data in mind.

15. Seventy-two women actually answered this question. Final questionnaire respondents who were sexually inactive were asked to skip it. Those who answered it were offered a choice not given on the original questionnaire, that of "nobody" (in addition to "myself," "my man," and "us both"). We added this option so that women would not be forced into saying "both" when condom use actually hadn't been negotiated. Eighteen in forty-seven respondents chose "nobody." Note that "my man" was used because participants typically used it in real speech.

16. While questionnaire responses indicate that the decision-making process is paramount, they also indicate that the categories provided were too broad. Data on perceived motivations, the imposition of unilaterally conceived plans, intentions, and circumstances, and conversations regarding condoms are sorely needed.

17. 442 men also participated in this study (Geringer et al. 1993). Of these, 46 percent of the 354 who reported ever having used condoms said that the decision was theirs; 37 percent said that the decision was joint; 17 percent said that their partners made the decision.

18. Penny, who had just left her husband of seven years (a crack-cocaine addict who only recently had been released from jail), said, "I've picked his pockets . . . and a couple of times I needed to have him watch my son and we had broke up while I was working and basically we had to act like we're still going together. [Interviewer: 'What did you have to do?'] Had sex."

19. Sarah was one of the few interviewees who said that she didn't feel self-sufficient. However, she did not live off of a man's income; she lived with her grandmother. Furthermore, she was working toward independence and self-sufficiency. She explained, "My mother always taught me to be independent you know, get your own, have your own, do your own, do what you can. . . . Be your own self, you know, where you don't have to wake up with nobody complaining about this [and that]."

20. Because of its nature, this research collected women's self-reports of male bestowals rather than directly measuring the actual monthly dollar value of male contributions of cash and kind. Further, women's claims of independence were only indirectly confirmed. Gathering accurate income or resource allocation poses quite a challenge, partly because of the often illegal means by which people bring resources into their homes (e.g., working "under-the-table," earning more than the welfare department would allow without cutting one's benefits, or even selling drugs). This notwithstanding, since women's perceptions do affect their behavioral choices whether or not these perceptions accurately reflect material reality, reliance on self-reports is not in itself a problem. In fact, self-reports reveal patterns objective measurements cannot expose. However, direct measurements of women's material realities should be gathered in the future so that a more precise model of the interplay between cultural ideals and women's real financial conditions may be developed.

21. Ostentatious display of male offerings sends other messages too, such as those concerning a woman's skill in catching successful men who support her well. The material benefits of conjugal relations do not detract from their affective worth which, in part due to culture and (unless prostitution is concerned) is paramount in the context of sex (as informants' discourse showed).

22. These findings may reflect a selection bias that affected Dayse's choice of women to approach regarding being interviewed (her response rate was 100 percent: all women asked to do so participated); however, I suspect that they do not. Dayse's overtly stated criteria for selection were a woman's presence in the clinic and her availability and her relationship status.

Chapter 7
The Psychosocial Benefits of Unsafe Sex

Sexual knowledge-sharing.

Motivation to share sex knowl = ↓HIV spread

This chapter uses study findings to show that unsafe sex is part of a psychosocial strategy for maintaining one's status and sense of self—a strategy that involves telling patterned narratives (as regarding a partner's faithfulness) and acting out scripts (as by engaging in unsafe sex) that optimistically confirm the quality of one's choice of a partner and so of one's relationship with him. Economic motives do, in some cases, play a role in encouraging some women's unsafe sex (e.g., Campbell 1990; Ward 1993a; Worth 1989) but, as Chapter 6 showed, purely materialist or economic approaches to urban minority women's risk-taking are inadequate (cf. Kline et al. 1992).

Such approaches ascribe the sex-related profit seeking motivations of many inner-city prostitutes or sex workers to all inner-city minority women, despite the fact that sex workers comprise only a small portion of inner-city female populations. Moreover, they disregard women's own testimony about their self-sufficiency, the high rate of unemployment among inner-city men of color, and the fact that inner-city men can and do seek and receive money from girlfriends (Weinberg and Williams 1988; Liebow 1967). In addition to these flaws, materialist models of inner-city heterosexual coupling may be further diminished by the relative sizes of condom using and non-using women's paychecks (these were bigger, on average, for non-users in this study), and the relative amounts of money that users and non-users receive from men (these were lower, on average, for non-users). Findings from this research suggest that emotional and sociocultural factors are more important determinants of most Black inner-city women's condom use decisions than financial considerations are.

The connotations of condoms, which implicate users as philanderers and carriers of disease, need not be confronted if condoms are not used.

Emotions/sociocultural factors limit impact of knowledge.

This chapter shows how, through barrierless sexual contact, women assure themselves that their relationships are committed, close, and intact, for only women with faithful partners have the freedom to have condomless sex. Unsafe sex provides women — particularly those dependent on relations with men for status and self-esteem — with a way to feel good about their lives (cf. Worth 1989).

The emotional and social dependence of women on men is promoted through heterosexual relationship ideals and the status and self-esteem considerations linked to these ideals. It seems to be associated also with the shape of women's immediate social networks and the style of their conjugal unions. Women with jealous partners appear to be more dependent on their men for emotional and social resources, as their social circles are kept small by and for the men. Such women seem to focus more on their conjugal relationships than do women who have larger social networks[1] and less jealous partners; therefore they may tend to engage in more wishful thinking about honest monogamy. This, in turn, may facilitate and depend on high levels of AIDS-risk denial and the practice of unsafe sex.

Before discussing the study women and the ideals affecting them, I must mention some suggestive findings about the women's perceptions of men's condom-use patterns. Only about one in five of the eighteen first-phase interviewees believed that the majority of men would agree to use a condom if asked to do so.[2] Just over three in five were sure that most men would refuse, by casting the woman as the HIV carrier ("Why? Do *you* have AIDS?"), by trying to talk her into believing that he could not be infected, by lying that, as one focus-group participant said, "I have some in my pocket" and then later claiming to have been mistaken, or by just saying "No." (Note that these attitudes and actions were attributed to men in general and not to any woman's particular male partner.)

Unsafe sex might provide some men a way to dominate women who are bold enough to ask for condom use (cf. Anderson 1990, 118–20; Worth 1990). Refusing to use condoms and so claiming dominance over women (and, for believers in a genocide plan, over whites) appears important for Black men, as racism, poverty, and poor education means that few other avenues to masculine self-esteem are open. W. Penn Handwerker (1993) notes that, among Black men in Barbados, non-use of condoms is related to perceived disempowerment and the desire to inflict abuse on women. More research into this is clearly needed; we know little regarding the ways in which these male perceptions and desires are played out in the U.S. sexual arena. We do know, however, what many women desire of men, as the next section shows.

Conjugal Factors

Heterosexual Relationship Ideals

As I argued in Chapter 2, many Black women idealize faithful monogamy, as do U.S. women in general. While Blacks may favor marrying later than whites do and condone single parenthood (Pittman et al. 1992), the two groups hold the same basic ideals for heterosexual relationships (see Anderson 1990; Cochran 1989; Oliver 1989; Stack 1974; see also Pivnick 1993). These include sexual and emotional fidelity. Most Black women look on other women who accept male infidelity with pity and scorn (Fullilove et al. 1990).

Interestingly, although the church is a very powerful institution in most Black communities (e.g., Worth 1990), clinic focus group participants responding to a question about whether religion affects condom use said, "No, it don't. Religion don't say [no to condoms] — it says to you to have one man, a mate," and "Religion stops you from having extramarital affairs outside the relationship but it doesn't have anything [to do with using condoms]." Indeed, despite the church's power, Blacks seem to be more interested in condoms than whites (to some degree, this reflects contraception method access and economic factors).

For example, findings from a survey of women attending family planning clinics indicate that Black women are more likely than white women to endorse condom use (Valdiserri et al. 1989). In a different study, one of male and female urban heterosexuals at risk for AIDS, Catania et al. (1993) found that, while 11 percent of white women claimed to use condoms "always," 14 percent of Black women did so. A similar difference emerged among men.[3] Moreover, the (modest) trend toward increased consistent condom use, identified through a comparison of these data with data collected in an earlier phase of the research, was particularly apparent among Blacks.[4]

While Black women may idealize monogamy, the cultural expectation that men will have multiple sex partners (cf. Fullilove et al. 1990; Liebow 1967) and the high rates of homicide, unemployment, and incarceration for inner-city males causes a scarcity of "good" men. In light of this shortage, many women choose to build families without the perceived burden of a husband or boyfriend drawn from the remainders (Wilson 1987). But, despite the fact that racist and other social and cultural conditions that contradict the monogamy imperative make most women's achieving it near impossible, belief in what Elijah Anderson calls "the dream" of faithful monogamy does persist; it is promoted through television soap operas, popular songs, and women's magazines (1990, 113–

The dream prevents knowledge from Δ behavior.

17). Accordingly, attaining "the dream" or even a close approximation brings prestige (cf. Mays and Cochran 1988).

For most M&I clinic clients, as for other urban Black women (e.g., Mays and Cochran 1988), cultural ideals regarding heterosexual relations make committed unions with men essential for achieving status and attaining happiness. Sex is an integral aspect of conjugal relations. Sometimes it can be unpleasurable. Peg, who is thirty-four and has two children, said that "especially after I had the baby he wanted to have sex in my butthole, my rectal, and I hated that and I never wanted him to do it. He would sneak into it and pin me down." Betsy's boyfriend of six years once asked her over the phone "to go to bed with all his friends. I told him 'No'." Her boyfriend got angry but later apologized "and he said that he needed me." For most women, however, and even in most cases for women who had experienced a negative incident(s), sex was a good thing involving much pleasure and little pressure.

Twenty-four-year-old Falasha, a pregnant mother of an eight-year-old boy, said that sex with her boyfriend is "sort of like we have a conversation, like a 'Do you like this?' kind of thing. So there will be sort of things like we would have a conversation and carry [them] out." Donna said that her partner will "say something like, 'I can understand a woman's body. I know that it's going to probably get sore.' So he says, 'So, how does it feel?' He asks me that stuff." "The sex, it's great you know and all," said twenty-one-year-old Sarah, who continued, "He never pushed me."

Bernice's partner, who was older, asked her to carry out a few non-traditional sexual actions but, she said, "I didn't feel comfortable 'cause I never did it before. It didn't cause any confusion. He didn't get angry. He was like, 'Whatever [you] feel comfortable with, that's what you are to do.'" Bernice continued, saying, "Sometimes I didn't [think I satisfied him sexually] but he always said he was." Sexual encounters with steady partners were, for the most part then, reported to be enjoyable.

Finding time and space for sex can be challenging in the inner city. Like many clinic clients, Shelly lives with family members. So when she and her partner want privacy, like many couples without a place to withdraw to, they go to a hotel. If they want to use condoms, they might stop off at a corner shop on the way; alternately, someone will bring supplies. Upon arrival at the hotel, many couples shower before settling into a romantic evening. Generally, showers are for hygienic rather than sexual purposes. As Mary explained, "That was just for our own protection. I want to kiss all over him and I want him to kiss all over me." Asked if she and her partner showered together, Mary responded, "No! Take your own, baby! I don't want that! My eyes are clean as soul: they don't [i.e., I'm not] open to that."

Shelly told me how she and her boyfriend first came to have sex:

Two months after we was together we was talking and, you know, I kissed him and he kissed me. We just felt — all of a sudden we were hooked up and we [realized we] were gonna go too fast . . . He waited about two weeks afterward and then I said "Oh well, let's go to the hotel." And he was like, "For real?" And I was like, "Sure." He was like, "Do you really — it's only if you really willing and ready to do it; I mean I'm not gonna push you or anything." And I was like, "OK. I want to go," and I did — I wanted to go. So we went and we made love and everything went just fine.

Sex can be just plain lustful, but as Janet, a single mother of seven children aged two through seventeen and a community college student who hoped to be a teacher, explained, women often have sex to "feel loved, needed, wanted." Janet also pointed out that with unsafe sex there is "nothing in between you both physically and emotionally. You are the closest to him that you can be." The emotional aspect of condom use is paramount for Janet and for many women who do not like the way that condoms feel.

"I guess it just feels like a lot of rubber in between us," said Rose, who had lived with her boyfriend for five years. When asked if she meant that the physical feeling of the rubber bothered her or if she meant something else, Rose replied, "Well, mental thing. It was more of a mental thing." Similarly, Falasha, who was pregnant and was using condoms "for safety of the baby," said that her dislike of condoms was "just a mental thing, you know, and not really — it's a mental thing but I can't get it to feel good." With the mental or emotional component of condom use in mind, the following statement by a focus group participant about how good sex with condoms can feel physically and her addendum about her preference to forgo them makes perfect sense:

First, I want to say they do have these really good condoms. No, really, these condoms are so good, I'm telling you. They're kinda expensive though. You will not know — I couldn't tell that he had one on. But secondly, I would prefer not to use them.

In response to an open-ended question about the advantages of not using condoms, almost half the women interviewed in the first phase of the research brought up the issue of trust. Condomlessness was directly described as "a sign of trust" and of "honesty" and "commitment." It was seen as "more romantic . . . special." One woman said, "It makes me feel like the relationship is strong and healthy and trustworthy and faithful"; another reported, "We feel closer to each other without condoms."

The frequency of spontaneous talk of trust among first-phase interviewees was surprisingly high in light of the noted question's tone and placement in the interview schedule (after a question about how condoms work), indicating the importance of the trust-related aspect of condom symbolism. Other data from the study suggest that the frequency of what I call "trust-talk" among the first-phase interviewees would have been much greater — perhaps 100 percent — had a question about trust been posed directly. So second-phase (clinic) interviewees were asked specifically about the qualities they desired in men as well as about how they felt about condoms.

Shelly, who had only recently been released from prison, declared, "If I can't trust my man than who can I trust? You know what I'm saying?" If a woman wants to be able to justify being with a particular man, she must feel able to say that he is trustworthy. Bernice, who at twenty-four had a five-year-old daughter, explained, "If you question a person a lot that means that you don't trust them and that's bad. [If you] can't trust each other, you ain't got no relationship, 'cause [relationships are] based on trust." Twenty-one-year-old Sarah had the same opinion: "Trust is the whole thing in a relationship, trust and honesty. If there is no trust, there is no honesty; there's no relationship."

Trust came up also in the context of condom use itself. Betsy, who was having troubles with her partner, told of an incident in which her man came to her for sex while having an affair: "I didn't trust him so I asked him to use a condom. He didn't want to, because he told me to trust him." Non-use of condoms demonstrates that trust has been established, as Peg's testimony shows: "When I first met [my partner] I used them 'til I really felt secure that he wasn't having sex with other people, and I didn't push the issue that much, but sometimes I would. I'd say, 'Better get your friend out of the drawer right there.' "

It often is noted in the literature on condom use that using condoms announces that partners are not sexually exclusive and signals a lack of mutual trust. This is made clear in the following interchange reported by a clinic focus group participant:

I went to my physical and everything and they told me that it was best that I started using rubbers . . . So I went and told my old man. I said, "Look, we have to start using rubbers" over the phone, and he said, "Well, I haven't done anything with anyone but you since we've been together."

Her "old man" responded as if in asking him to use condoms the woman had accused him of infidelity.

The strength of the association between condoms and extraconjugal sex means that condom use denotes failure in a relationship. Josephine, a first-phase focus group participant with one young son had been with her partner for over five years. Despite the fact that he infected her with gonorrhea three years prior to the project, Josephine's belief in her partner's current faithfulness was high and she saw no need for condoms: "I know my man ain't, you know, doing this and that [i.e., cheating]." Clinic interviewee Linda, who had been married five years, said, "I don't worry about [condoms] because my husband, as far as I know, has been faithful to me, and I believe he is, so I don't worry about it."

Because of condoms' connotations, even simply having them on hand can cause problems. Interviewee Mary said, "If you're honest to him, what do you need them for?" Later, in defining honesty, Mary equated it with the word monogamy. Like Mary, Peg felt that she did not need condoms. Still, she had "a drawer full of them [from the clinic]. He counts [them] some days to see if I have other lovers." Clarissa was the suspicious one in her relationship: "I found one in the glove compartment and he [suggested that] maybe I put it in there, and I'm like, 'Oh, right.' I ripped it right open and [punched a hole in it as he looked on. And I said] 'I don't appreciate you accusing me.'" She asked him rhetorically, "What is this for? You know, I'm going in your pocket when I wash your clothes and finding them." The implication that her partner has extraconjugal sex was clear to her.

Betsy's partner sometimes had condoms when he came to see her but he never used them with her. Rather than talking about how this might have meant that he had been cheating, she asserted that "he just had them to show off to his friends, so they could see that he was doing things, I guess," she said, adding once more, "He had to show off." Showing off about cheating and actually doing so are two different things, she suggested.

Nicole told a story about her boyfriend "trying to wear a condom to really piss me off, because we had been together for so long." This statement's intelligibility to the listener depends on his or her having knowledge of the connotations condoms carry, which Nicole made explicit as she went on. She and her partner had broken up and one day he came home looking for love:

We was kissing and doing our love, and I had no clothes on and he had no clothes on and he was like, "Wait a minute" [while he got a condom]. He was really pissing me off, but I hid it 'cause I was just like "Oh, OK," you know. He's just trying to make me think like he was with somebody, 'cause we was totally away from each other. . . . It's games. He like to play mind games.

Marvelle tells a similar story, speaking from the opposite position: "Sometimes [I] want to aggravate him, so I'll get him and say, 'Here, you gotta use this [condom] cause I don't know where you've been,' and there's an argument you know, [him saying] 'What do you mean, I have been good, what [are] you thinking?'" In telling this story, Marvelle made the assertion that implying that one's partner is untrustworthy (adulterous) is a cunning way to annoy him. Importantly, she was not saying that her partner actually did have affairs. In fact, just seconds prior to telling the story, Marvelle said, "I'll only believe that he doesn't."

Women generally prefer to ignore their men's shortcomings when they can because without partners women are subject to shortages of emotional and social resources. Manlessness can leave women feeling unloved or lonely, and it can lower their self-esteem and status. So women actively use unsafe sex to demonstrate to themselves that their men do not stray sexually. They do so as part of a psychosocial strategy for building and preserving an image of themselves as having achieved the conjugal ideal.

Women can build status and self-esteem by presenting themselves to others as having attracted loyal, honorable partners and as having attained perfect, intact unions. They commonly pattern stories about their relationships with men on either or both of two narrative forms, the "Monogamy Narrative" and the "Wisdom Narrative." The latter involves claims of having used wisdom in making partner choices; the former involves claims of having an excellent and monogamous relationship.

Unsafe Sex and the "Wisdom Narrative"

The main reason that women engage in unsafe sex has less to do with economics than with condom symbolism and women's social and affective needs, which include the needs for status and esteem. In fact, an active distaste for instrumentally motivated sex informs condom use decisions: a woman who uses condoms is likened to (or is) a prostitute. Prostitutes or sex workers are said to use condoms with each customer. Their sexuality appears unrelated to any desire to establish or maintain long-term relationships. But even prostitutes tend to practice unsafe sex with boyfriends and husbands because, even to prostitutes, condoms imply a social distance and a profit motive that is inappropriate in the context of an existing — or a potentially existing — personal relationship (Miller et al. 1990, 260–61; see also Sibthorpe 1992).

Most women want to establish long-term relationships that meet the standards entailed in heterosexual relationship ideals. Women know that, in light of these ideals, to achieve and maintain self-respect and the respect of others they must first of all be able to determine the past sexual (and IV drug) histories and the present intentions of men. Then, they must act accordingly. I call talk and action that supports a belief in one's own ability to identify "clean" (disease-free) and "conscious" (honorable) men or that advertises this ability to one's peers the "Wisdom Narrative."

Unsafe sex is an essential element in the Wisdom Narrative. An unattached woman engaging in casual sex maintains the beliefs that her ability to judge men is well developed and that her standards for partners are high by not using condoms, for to use them would—except in certain contexts soon discussed—be to label herself as a careless harlot and an unintelligent person who cannot tell a "good" man from a "bad" one. A woman's insistence on condoms casts her partner as diseased and so of poor quality and certainly not steady boyfriend or husband material. One focus group participant described a scenario in which a high school student tossed the condoms ("safeties") passed out to her and the other students in her health class to a friend, teasing, "You need these more than me. You're messing with Joe, and you don't know *what* he has."

Condom use shows that a man cannot be trusted, despite his claim to be "clean," and despite his claims to respect and love whichever woman he may go home with that night. Even a casual liaison with such a man is not esteemed, for while a man may have sex with a woman purely for gratification, and despite her ultimate "badness" or "goodness," a double standard is held whereby women are expected to seek stable relationships and so should only have sex with men seen as fit to be involved with conjugally. A woman's ability to spot and deal wisely with (i.e., avoid) men who are sweet-talking "[game] players"—and so potential HIV carriers—is essential.

According to participants, men say anything to have condomless sex (regarding men and sex-procurement related lies, see Cochran 1989). Many women reported that men will say that they do not enjoy sex with condoms when such is not the case simply so that they do not have to bother with the condoms. In addition to the typical coercive laments regarding "feeling," men tell women that they are "clean" and not involved with any other women. But, as clinic focus group women said, "They're going to lie. They don't want to tell a woman what they done did," and "They lie, 'cause that's a man."

In an extended statement on male lying, made in relation to men in general but also with her children's father in mind, Adrienne explained:

Well, men say they don't have no other woman or lady friends, and a man is a liar about staying with his family, taking care of his family, where he'll go out in the streets and take care of another family. He lies about sexual things. The man will give you a disease and tell a lie and beat you up and say you gave him the disease. A man is just a liar, he's a born liar.

Earlier, in regard to this ex-partner, I had asked her, "Did you love him?" Adrienne replied, "Yeah, very much. I still do."

As far as condoms go, men may tell women that they use them with all the others so there is no need to worry, or that they just got out of prison and have not had sex for many years (that incarcerated men may have sex

with men remains unsaid). The sincerity of some such promises notwithstanding, it is very painful for women to admit that the men they are
intimate with may lie and possibly even use them as sex objects. "Other"
men may lie, but acknowledging a particular, chosen partner's duplicity
by using condoms could force a woman to experience her decision to
undertake intercourse as stupid or unwise and so as humiliating.

So, despite male tale-telling, women often assume that the men they
themselves would have sex with are truthful — and true (cf. Kinsey 1994).
In response to another focus group participant's request for condom
users to raise their hands, and perhaps because she knew that the project's aim was condom use promotion, one woman asked, "How many of
us sit here and take the risk? We got educated. You [a staff member]
educated us. We sat here and [you] gave out the rubbers. Who used
them? The same as we talk to a crowd of friends, and say 'Girl, you better
use some rubbers —'" The woman was cut off by another participant,
who declared, "You haven't used none with the three guys you've been
with." Following some good-natured banter about the number of men
implicated (a failed ploy to change the subject), the woman responded,
"No, I did not use them; I did not raise my hand."

Women may "take the risk" of condomless sex because condom use
would undermine their claims to having chosen partners wisely. That is,
unsafe sex can be preferable to ruining one's self-esteem and perceived
social standing. One's AIDS risk can be denied through the very acting
out of Wisdom Narratives, in unsafe sex (as it can through the telling of
these narratives, to oneself and to others). In addition to its role in dem-
onstrating one's wisdom, unsafe sex with a date or a not-yet-permanent
partner demonstrates one's desire to establish that partner's perma-
nency (cf. Pivnick 1993); through unsafe sex he has been deemed worthy,
and a committed, stable, monogamous conjugal relationship — a relationship true to the model that this culture recommends — is shown to be
the goal.

Long-Term Relationships and the "Monogamy Narrative"

The Wisdom Narratives of women who define themselves as involved
in long-term relationships (rather than as single or dating) are contained within a larger narrative form which I call the "Monogamy Narrative." This narrative describes an idealized, monogamous, heterosexual
union — the kind of union that participants feel brings the most status
and esteem (see Worth 1990; also see Wilson 1987 regarding choosing
not to attempt such unions, in which case, perhaps, Wisdom Narratives
suffice). Both male manipulations, like making promises not intended
for keeping, and the popular heterosexist discourse on coupling commu-

nicated by the media and by female peers fuel belief in this American dream (see Anderson 1990, 113–17).

Research participants (and visiting males in the first-phase focus groups) often stated that "men are dogs" who eagerly cheat on their main conjugal partners. Findings from the literature lend support to the contention that men are adulterous. At least one in three unmarried but cohabiting urban American men who participated in a study by Blumstein and Schwartz had extraconjugal sex (cited in Turner et al. 1989, 111). Nearly 40 percent of unmarried Black men between the ages of eighteen and forty-five have multiple partners (Bower 1991).[5] However, because admitting that one's partner has sex with other women damages "self-pride" and social position, women in unions deny infidelity by telling Monogamy Narratives, proclaiming that their men, and so their relationships, are ideal. Like the Wisdom Narrative it subsumes, the Monogamy Narrative involves implicit, self-congratulatory comparisons to other women's rocky conjugal relations; it is infused with Neil Weinstein's "optimistic bias" (1989).

The optimistic bias was implicit in statements from clinic focus group women responding to a fellow participant's above-mentioned request for a show of hands by those who did use condoms. As if speaking for the group, one woman said, "I don't use nothing with [my baby's father] 'cause we're not cheating." Another woman told the others that she did not need condoms with her partner because he "hasn't done anything with anyone but me." Someone asked her, "How long have you been together?"

"About a year and a half, but when I met him he was a celibate."

"He told you he was celibate?"

"Yeah, he was celibate; he didn't mess around."

"Well I don't know and you don't know, but if he says so, fine."

The insult in the last statement was partly provoked by the first woman's unspoken claim that her partner is cut from better or at least different cloth than most men. While the ability to see optimistic biases in one's own statements and actions (e.g., condomless sex with a self-proclaimed "celibate") is rare, women often can see them in others'. This was implicit in the aforementioned assertion that "the same as we talk to a crowd of friends, and say 'Girl, you better use some rubbers' [we don't use them ourselves]."

Clarissa, the woman who at one point in her interview at the clinic told me that she found condoms in the glove compartment and in her partner's pocket, said optimistically at a later point that she did not think he was seeking sex from an outside source. "Uh-uh," she said; "No. But if he does — I don't think so, cause he loves me. He wouldn't." However, she

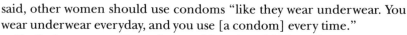

said, other women should use condoms "like they wear underwear. You wear underwear everyday, and you use [a condom] every time." Similarly, non-user Dee, who was thirty-six, said of condoms:

I recommend everyone use them now. [When] I have friends that are going out with somebody, I give them three or four and make sure they put them in their purses. I have nothing against them at all. I'm one-hundred percent behind them . . . I say, "Well, it's better to be uncomfortable for a few minutes than have AIDS for the rest of your life." ["But in your relationship you don't?"] No, I don't use them.

I said to Dee, "You don't think they're necessary?" and she said, "As far as I believe in my relationship, I don't think so. But as far as anyone else just starting up with someone, yeah."

Like Clarissa and Dee, Linda explained that she did not use condoms because her partner was faithful. She then went on to say,

I don't worry about [condom use] for myself, but I see all these people out here [i.e., at the clinic] and they don't realize how close it is. They think it can't happen to them and it really can. That's what my friend, who is married to this man that is cheating on the side — it bothers me.

Linda had previously explained,

[Her husband] had like about five venereal diseases in the last five months and he hasn't gave her any but still, I told her, "As quick as he can give you those, he can give you AIDS. I think that you love somebody who is just throwing your life away as well as theirs, you know, and who's gonna be there to raise your child?"

Linda also said, "I have a lot of friends who are married and it's like, I wouldn't want to be married to their spouses, not at all. They're cheating or they not spending any time, or they want to do what they want to do and my husband is not like that. I have to give him a lot of credit."

To maintain Monogamy Narratives, women engage in unsafe sex; safer-sex would signal infidelity (regarding female IDUs in particular, see Pivnick 1993 and Sibthorpe 1992). Gloria, a focus group participant, said, "If my husband came to me and handed me some condoms, I think I'd shoot him because I'd know then that he's out there doing something that he ain't got no business doing." Likewise, women who introduce condoms themselves can imply that they have been unfaithful: another focus group participant said, "If she just comes out of the blue with something like that, he might think *she's* messing around."[6] A woman in the clinic focus group patiently explained this to the researcher present: "Well, they think that you're going to have sex with some other man, honey, like you got some kind of infections." Someone added,

"When they first see them, they're mad." Condoms' negative connotations regarding a woman's sex life also were invoked through interviewee Nicole's self-saluting claim, "They're not necessary, 'cause I'm just with one man."

In any case, few women said that they would ask their partners to use condoms. Because women have faith in the conjugal ideal and because their status is partly based on the loyalty and other qualities of their mates, a double standard exists by which all men except one's own are bound to "mess around." As in the simpler Wisdom Narratives, generic men and one's own man are held in mind separately so that cognitive processes do not bring them into contact and expose their similar tendencies. The same woman who declares, "A man is going to be a man" and advises other women to be sure to use condoms will boast, "I got a *good* man," using claims about her relationship to impress her family and friends. As focus-group participants said, "They want to believe the best," and "They want to *trust* that person — to feel that they can *trust* them."

A clinic focus group participant recognized the dangers of such wishful thinking and warned that "In every walk of life there's a man out there screwing around, and that's what we as women have to look at. Don't think 'cause my man is in this category here, he doesn't mess around." That is, he does. But, as a woman in the same group explained, "If you are married or whatever and you have been with a person for twelve years or whatever, you automatically assume you've been faithful to one another and then if the issue comes up, then 'What do we need a condom for?' 'I ain't been with nobody.' "

To find out more about women's alleged propensity to "automatically assume" and to "want to believe the best," we asked the eighteen first-phase interviewees how they would feel when confronted with the news that their men had been cheating. All men may be "dogs," but only two interviewees (11%, N = 18) would immediately believe the acquaintance's report. Five (27.8%) would deny the message's truth by contending that the women their partners were seen with were business associates, old friends, family members, or otherwise innocent relations. Six (33.3%) of the eighteen women would doubt the messenger's motives. They explained that a devious woman may try to secure another's man by telling her that he was cheating; a man may try to secure a woman's affections by maligning her current partner.

Ten of the interviewees (55.6%, N = 18) said that they would ask their partners about the sightings eventually if not at first but, in the words of one focus group participant, "You kind of overlook things, you know. You find excuses to not believe." Participants described the female tendency to deny the reality of adultery much as Elijah Anderson describes female partner idealization and male manipulation in a hypothetical poor, young, urban pair:

> The girl's faith in the dream clouds her view of the situation . . . Until she completely loses confidence in him, she may find herself strongly defending the young man to friends and family who question her choice . . . Aware of many abandoned young mothers, many a girl fervently hopes that her man is the one who will be different. (1990, 115–16)

Many women believe that they will be able to tell if their partners are indeed cheating. In the context of a focus group discussion of condoms and male cheating, one woman said, "I don't use them at all with my man, I think he'd tell me if—I'd notice when he had—" Another participant cut her off: "You can't risk that." In other words, "you might not know or guess that he was cheating and you should not take that chance." But women do take such chances, because, as the first speaker said, "Well, I think I [would] know." Clues include shifts in partners' sexual preferences, changes in their visiting patterns, and changes in the frequency with which they want to have sex. As interviewee Dee said, "I probably know just about how often he like to have sex, and if [it changes] then I know, see."

Even so, women do not always know—or believe—that their partners are having affairs. As a staff member who popped in on the clinic focus group said to the participants,

> A lot of young ladies come in who have STDs and they come back and they say, "He says he don't have it." I say, "Have you been unfaithful to him?" and they say "No, I haven't been unfaithful." I says, "You sit here telling me that you know you haven't been outside the relationship but you know that that man is telling you you've got this out of thin air?" And they will take that in, but they say "But I love him."

Interviewee Mary explained that often it was not out of "thin air" that one got such diseases: "You get infections from wearing tampons; you get infections from wearing panties."

When monogamy is the ideal, a man's unfaithfulness brings hurt feelings: "You kind of know [about his extraconjugal affairs] and you don't want to face it because you know it's going to hurt your heart," said focus-group participant Ernestine, who had experienced such with her current partner. Partners' affairs also bring shame, especially to women who publicly boast of their men's faithfulness. Disinclined to experience pain or lose status, women deny the possibility of adultery in their relationships. Condomlessness helps them do this as it implies fidelity.

Women know that suggesting condom use can hurt their partners' feelings because of condoms' connotations, and so some women threaten to punish men's adultery with forced condom use, increasing the negative symbolic load that condoms carry (cf. Fullilove et al. 1990). Punishment, if enacted, lasts only for a few days: the time that it takes for the man to cleanse his body of the sexual fluids and essence left behind by the other woman (or man). While empowering for women, the emphasis on punishment and hygiene masks the long-term possibilities of disease transmission and so is self-defeating.[8]

 As important as it is, infidelity is not the only negative message condoms convey. There are other forms of duplicity associated with their use. Some participants said that men secretly poke pin-holes in condoms so that they can impregnate women (see also Jones 1991; Sobo 1993b). Larger holes let a man "feel the flesh" without latex in the way while the woman thinks that the condom, which she saw being put on, is protecting her (and him).

Fear and Altruistic Compliance

The strength of condoms' negative connotations and the power of women's denial was clearly expressed during a focus group discussion in which the possibility was raised of showing pregnant women photos of babies and children with AIDS in order to convince them to practice safer sex. Evoking fear while offering information on risk-reduction's effectiveness and while mobilizing concerns about spreading HIV to significant others had been shown to hold some promise for motivating risk reduction behavior (see Turner et al. 1989, 266–68, 279; Tunstall et al. 1991) and the M&I AIDS education director devised the sick baby scheme in light of this.

 Participants liked the idea of scare tactics. In fact, even before we broached the photo idea, many focus group participants suggested that educators should use "scary-ass" pictures or films that show the physical devastation that AIDS involves. One participant thought that bringing in an extremely good-looking HIV-positive individual would be useful, as people would realize that they would easily have had condomless sex — and perhaps even have purposefully conceived babies — with this attractive person. Others agreed.

Those who saw the photos were visibly shaken by the suffering and wastage depicted. But in discussion participants said that most women would claim, "Hell, my baby won't look like that. My baby has a good daddy. And this daddy doesn't mess around — he only messes with *me*." A typical response to this kind of claim was, "Well, honey, that's what *you* think. I just saw him over at Gloria's house, and it was more than a social call he was making."

Refusing to acknowledge the possibility that one's mate has sex with other women (or men) supports the Monogamy Narrative. Unsafe sex supports it too: unsafe sex deflects attention from adultery and deceit and focuses it instead on the trust and honesty. It helps women maintain the belief that theirs are monogamous, caring, satisfying unions that leave neither partner desirous of sex or love from outside sources, as is prescribed by the popular U.S. conjugal ideal.

Before moving on I must mention that in addition to trusting one another, partners in conjugal unions are expected to feel compassion for one another. Earlier, I noted that many women doubt men's claims that condom use reduces their sexual pleasure. However, some believe that such is true. Nicole said, "I know that they don't like them. If you're going to have sex with somebody and know they really don't prefer rubbers . . ." Nicole did not finish expressing this thought, but the implication that a woman who forced a partner who did not like condoms to use them was an uncaring woman indeed seemed quite clear. A lack of compassion would be just as out of place as a condom in an ideal conjugal relationship.

Safer Casual Sex and the "Alternative Wisdom Narrative"

The Wisdom Narrative and the Monogamy Narrative both hold strong sway over the ways in which sexuality and condom use are (and are not) actualized. However, there are exceptions to the rules. Some women do practice safer sex despite the cultural pressures against it. While safer sex generally implies that one needs to protect oneself from one's partner and so suggests that one's partner is not of high quality, an alternative interpretation exists. In certain circumstances, and if one represents one's choice to use condoms very carefully both to oneself and to others, practicing safer sex can be considered very wise indeed.

If a woman in a long term relationship decides to have extraconjugal sex, condom use is considered judicious. Sara proclaimed, "If you cheat, wear a condom." Nicole said, "If I had more than one sexual partner, yeah I would wear a rubber. Yeah, I would wear them because I ain't taking no — If I was to like have an affair on my boyfriend or something like that, I would definitely use a rubber, hell yeah. . . . If that ever happened."

Nicole was not, at that time, involved in an affair. But, like men, some women do have multiple partners. Most Blacks think this disrespectable and so, according to participants, women often will deny that they do it.[9] Participants also said in passing that women who cheat tend to worry the most about their primary partners' infidelities because they project their own desires and behaviors onto their men. However, I found that the women who talked about secondary partners — and only a few of them did so—were generally separated from their men, often because of the men's incarceration. In any case, and as out of place as it is in a primary relationship, condom use was an expected accompaniment to outside or secondary affairs. This was in keeping with what I call the "Alternative Wisdom Narrative."

When talking about clinicians' propensity to hand out condoms, Vicki said, "I'll keep them and use them if I had to, if I had sex with somebody else." Recently, she had sex with a man who works at a nearby garage. "I just gave [him the condom] when we got to the hotel, 'cause you know it was gonna happen eventually," she said. Another time, she and another man "used three and then there weren't any more and the guy said, 'There ain't no more,' and I was all, 'That doesn't mean that you don't got to use one!' "

Mary, a straight-talking, smart, statuesque woman of thirty-six years who had only recently given up drugs, heartily endorsed the use of condoms, but she did not use them with her man. She wove the Alternative Wisdom Narrative and the Monogamy Narrative together in a manner that easily revealed her optimistic bias:

I think condoms period is good, no—excellent, 'cause they can prevent a lot of diseases and a lot of babies that are just not being taken care of and not being wanted. But I've been with this man for ten years. I know what he do and I know what I do. I have had no disease and no infections since I've been with this man, so that's why [we don't use condoms]. But if I do decide to leave this man, most definitely [the next] man will put a rubber on his tongue, his finger, and his penis. On his ear, on his face, on his head; 'cause I want it on . . . No, I don't need condoms. But if I'm with another man, I said he's going to be condomed down from head to toe, even his eyes, all over. Always use them, I don't care if I'm with you for two years, you got to have it.

I interrupted, "But in your particular circumstances with your boyfriend now?" Mary replied:

No I wouldn't, because I've known him, he knows me. Anybody else, sure, and I advise—'cause you don't know what nobody else be doing, you don't even know what you're doing. So you know you have to put a [condom] on that [penis]. I know [my partner] ain't doing nothing, but I'm screening [i.e., watching out] for another female, 'cause see sometimes their men have a whore, but I know my man, I know mine.

Later, in regard to sex with secondary partners who refuse to use condoms, Mary said,

If I tell a guy to put this on and he's gonna cuss me out, [I tell him] "You just don't need me. I don't know where you've been. Your body just looks good to me [and so] you think I can't do nothing [to stand up to you because I must have you]." My mama always told me that the penis is good, but the penis will get you in a lot of trouble like the diseases of today. And mama never lied . . . Uh-uh, I ain't doing that, girl. Even if a man [says he's] too big, I'll tell him, "I don't want none of that." . . . The penis is a big deal 'cause it can get you in very serious trouble."

How would she broach the topic of condom use with a new man or an extraconjugal partner? Mary told me that she would say, "I'll put this on and this is so we can both be sure about ourselves, not about that I think I'm cleaner than you or you cleaner than me. We want to protect each other." Within the context of a secondary or a new relationship, Mary made no bones about her feeling that "safety is very, very excellent."

Because an extraconjugal affair is not a primary relationship, condom use within one does not stir up the same issues that it does in a supposedly monogamous union. If conceptualized with care — if thought about without reference to particulars such as the possibly unsavory nature of one's partner but instead with reference to global statements like "you never know" or, as Mary said, "We want to protect each other" — condom use during extraconjugal intercourse indexes only that an affair is not a primary relationship, and that the participants are socially responsible in that they each have their primary partner's health interests in mind. Further, female adulterers act honorably to avoid making their primary partners into the unwitting sociological fathers of children conceived with other men. As one clinic focus group participant said, "If I had sex outside of my relationship, I don't know if I could really enjoy sex without it [a condom]"; she would be worrying about pregnancy or disease.

Without implicating their own partners, women explained that men who have sex outside their primary relationships are acting responsibly when using condoms, just as the women felt that they were acting responsibly when they practiced safer sex extraconjugally. One clinic focus group participant said, "I was with a guy on Saturday night and I told him to use a rubber and it didn't even faze him. He put it right on . . . He might have a wife or a woman at home. If he got the real deal at home, they getting the real thing, so every time they show a little respect." Using condoms with outside or secondary partners demonstrates respect for inside or primary partners. Further, condom use in the extraconjugal setting is justified or made tolerable by the fact that condoms are not used at home, where they do not belong.

Ordinarily, a woman will keep the general image of the responsible condom-using man separate from the particular image she has of her (loyal) primary partner. But in very special situations the two images can be allowed to overlap. For example, a focus group participant said, "My baby's father is in the Navy and I told him — you can't tell a man what to do. A man's gonna do what he wants to. And I told him — I gave him four rubbers and I said, 'Here, take this with you.' " The man's employment by the Navy and his related need to travel away from home made admitting his extraconjugal affairs in the context of talk about condom use a wise thing to do rather than humiliating (rhetorical statements about men in general also helped excuse this man's infidelities).

It is important to note that most women's circumstances would not, like the Navy wife's did, mitigate a man's infidelity. So most women talked of letting partners have (protected) outside sex in a general way, as in relation to other women or women in general and not in relation to themselves specifically. For instance, one woman in the same focus group said, "If you love him and are all infatuated with him, you probably would say 'OK, come on back here,' because you're in love—you're stupid"; note that the woman said "you," not "I." Interestingly, especially in light of the last chapter's discussion of materialist models of urban sexuality, while financial need ("the crunch down") was invoked a few times to explain why other women might allow themselves to be pressed into unsafe sex, participants were much more likely to attribute such submission to other women's lack of experience, love for partners, ignorance about partners' infidelities, or high-quality sex lives ("He make good love and she don't want to let that go").

A few women ended up in primary partnerships with men with whom they first used condoms, and like those who use condoms in secondary relationships, they justified their actions (which, of course, were no longer seen to be needed) by invoking the Alternative Wisdom Narrative. "When it's the beginning of a relationship I always use condoms, 'cause I don't know—with that last person, she might have AIDS as far as I know," said Sarah. "When it first started," said Peg, "I didn't want him to touch me. I was very scared of catching AIDS or herpes. I was scared." Although she "didn't push the issue," Peg asked her partner to use condoms for the first few months of their relationship. For her, as for Sarah, preliminary condom use was a sign of wisdom: "My father just died of AIDS for drug use, you know," she told me, "and it's not something that I want. I don't want to go out the door that way. And please, if he is fooling around with others, [he should] go on, leave me alone, please, please." Once trust was established, the women who wisely used condoms early on no longer saw them as necessary.

Unlike Peg and Sarah, Penny did not use condoms when her relationship began, but with the (alternative) wisdom of hindsight she said that she was not as smart as she should have been then: "He never really frightened me as much as I know [he] probably should have. . . . I never [used condoms] 'cause I loved him so much, I wasn't thinking."

Shelly, a twenty-three-year-old mother of one, told a story about a relationship that she wisely nipped in the bud:

I asked him if he would [use a condom] since it was going to be our first time. I said, "We need to use protection because I ain't having any sex with a man without using a rubber," and he said, "Well, I don't use one," and I said, "Well you can't — we can't be doing it." So he was like, "What you mean we can't?" And I said, "Take me back home 'cause if you can't use this then we have nothing in common." So he took me back home 'cause he refused to use them."

Safer Sex in Primary Relationships

While most talk of the wisdom of safer sex concerned secondary relationships (or temporary circumstances, as with the Navy wife and as with a new romance), and while condom-use rates among study participants were relatively low, some women did manage to use them on a fairly regular basis with long-term primary partners. For instance, six (24%) of the twenty-five clinic interviewees used condoms with their primary partners during their last sexual encounters (one other used condoms the last time that she had sex but this was with an outside partner; condom in this situation already has been discussed).

The reasons given for condom use with primary partners varied. Two of the women were primarily concerned about disease (both also used other contraceptive methods: pills for one, foam for the other). The third woman, a member of the Hebrew Israelite religion, used condoms to protect her child-to-be from toxins (including hormones) carried in semen and vaginal fluids (she said that she would probably continue to use them after the pregnancy for family planning purposes). The fourth and fifth used condoms primarily for birth control, and the sixth used them for both birth control and disease protection.

The latter woman, Bernice, was particularly wary of men. She was still very much in love with a partner who left her while she was in prison, although she was now in a new relationship. And, as she explained, "To tell you the truth, I'm not a sexually active person. I can do without, or I can have sex or I can — I really don't enjoy sex as much as some people do. I just don't get into it really, so it really doesn't bother me if I used them." Bernice seemed unhappy to me, and it may well be that her self-described asexual nature stemmed from a broken heart. The connotations of condoms as "safeties" or armor to protect women against men might have held special appeal to her. Indeed, when asked what she had heard about condoms, she came to their defense, explaining that a condom is "a protector." She went on, "It's just separating you all — separating your bodies from each other." The barrier image might have held special emotional resonance for Bernice, who was not in love with the man she was having sex with and desired to maintain her emotional distance from him.

Shelly, who used foam for birth control, used condoms "because it's a lot of things out here, lot of things. Strange things, you know, and AIDS." Sometimes she and her partner used two condoms (this may weaken the condoms because of excess friction between layers of latex): "You slam one on and then you slam another one on, to be extra-safe, extra-safe." Both Shelly and her partner, who "wants to be safe too" provided condoms, as seen in her description of the last time that they made love:

We just went in the store; he bought a rubber but I had already had one. He said, "We're going to the hotel," and I was like—we took showers and. . . . I handed him a rubber and he—he was like handing me one, and I was like, "So you're prepared," and he was like, "Yeah, I see you prepared too," and he—I put it on him and we got busy. We used both of them at the same time to make sure we was protected.

Shelly uses condoms " 'cause I love myself. I love myself and if I love myself I have to protect everything about me, you know: my body, my way of life." Here I must note that knowing people with AIDS does not seem to be related to condom use (cf. Pivnik 1993; Zimet 1992). For example, thirty-four-year-old Peg's father died of AIDS-related causes but she does not use condoms, because she feels "secure" about her partner's loyalty. While none of the condom-using interviewees referred to the loss of a loved one to AIDS as a motivating factor, self-protection and also self-respect figured importantly in the eyes of those who, like Shelly, used condoms to prevent disease.

Self-protection and self-respect figured also in some of the stories that participants told about other women who used, or who needed to use, condoms. A clinic focus group participant said,

I believe that if you love yourself with all these diseases coming out now you'll have respect for loving yourself and use a condom, especially if you're having many multiple partners. But if you just got one man and he ain't messing around, then you might not use them then, it depends on your relationship, if you have more than one sex partner.

Note that despite the importance of loving oneself, the advice to use condoms is diverted by a comparison between open and closed or so-called monogamous relationships which reflects the generally accepted wisdom that monogamy is an AIDS-proof type of arrangement. Shelly's ability to avoid such a diversion has to do with the fact that she is able to personalize the theory that men will stray without feeling threatened. Most women cannot do so.

Although she has plans for a future with her man, Shelly admits in reference not just to all men but also to her own that "a man's never committed totally. He's gonna mess around. So therefore, he — you choose to protect your own body, no matter if he ain't protecting his, you protect yours: you use condoms." And she did.

Shelly loved her partner but she did not worry about losing him: "When he ready to go, go ahead, you know." Perhaps with the exception of the two women who used condoms specifically to protect against disease, other participants did not share Shelly's idea that their partners would inevitably "mess around" on them but they did say things about losing men that were similar to what Shelly had to say. One focus-group participant said that she would leave a man herself if he threatened aggressively that he would abandon her if she refused to have condomless sex. Another explained, "Even though you love a guy, you can love a person to a certain degree. I don't care if it is your mate, it comes to a point — you love him [but] he's a man. He can be replaced. There's more men out there." Someone asked her about her own relationship, and she said,

I am in love with him, but I'm saying to a certain degree — he's got to give me some kind of respect, for my health and my safety . . . If he says he's going to go get another woman, he just has to go. I might be hurt, but that ain't gonna stop me [from holding my ground . . .] It doesn't mean I got to go along with what he do.

Someone in the group pressed the speaker for more information and she said, "Men are like busses; there's always another one coming." This kind of thinking may be related to condom use. In order to illuminate other factors that also may be related, let me return to my description of the condom-using interviewees.

I mentioned that Shelly and her partner both provided condoms. Falasha, who had "only had sex like five times" since conceiving because of a belief that it is not good for the development of the fetus, generally supplied her partner with condoms, and sometimes put them on him. She said, "I always have them, you know." Women may have easier access to condoms than many men because women visit clinics much more often due to their reproductive health needs and their childcare roles.

Michelle also supplied the condoms in her relationship, and their use was originally her idea. She requested that her partner wear condoms for contraception (she also used birth control pills), and "He was like, 'Yeah, I agree with you. We're not trying to start a family'." She recommended that to implement condom use "You should discuss it. You should discuss before you get ready to do the act, though. Discuss it over dinner, discuss it at the movies." "For me," she said, "I know what would happen and I think about the larger picture of what they have to pass these ten minutes

or these fifteen minutes and then I have to deal with the rest of my life."
And Michelle had plans for the rest of her life that included college and a
degree in social work.

As I listened to Michelle, it became obvious that her main reason for
wanting to use condoms had to do with protection against disease rather
than conception. Nevertheless, and importantly, by casting condoms as
needed for birth control, Michelle and other women who do so avoid
drawing their own or their partners' attentions to condoms' damning
connotations. Women who did not use condoms regularly also often
appealed to their role as contraceptives when explaining their occasional
use. Just after Clarissa had her baby, her partner came to her for sex. She
said, "I don't even get two or three weeks [rest] and he was like, 'I want
some now,' you know. Well, OK. So I told him, 'Well, OK, I'm gonna give
you this box [of condoms]. . . . Here you're gonna use these 'cause I
don't want no more children, no more.' "

Another strategy for diverting attention from the negative symbolic
load that condoms can carry involved appealing to sexual pleasure. Indeed, the first time that Clarissa and her partner even used a condom,
they did so " 'cause we never used one before, and I never had, you
know. . . . [It was] like a thrill thing." She said, "I had them 'cause I
had just had [my baby] and they give you birth-control pills, foam, and
rubbers — a box of twelve — so you know, [you] just have them around the
house."

The enhancement condoms add to sex can go beyond the "thrill
thing" of novelty. One woman, a clinic focus group participant, said, "I

suggest to him the same thing that you [attending clinic staff member]
suggested to me. You said that the rubbers will make him last longer, and
it worked. I tried it." Her experience indicates that sex-positive education
messages can be quite effective.

Here, I must note that for some women there comes a point when a
man's condom-enhanced ability to "last longer" becomes unenjoyable.
Donna, an interviewee who felt no need for condoms as her partner had
tested negative for HIV antibodies and as he was not "messin' around
with nobody," said that what she "didn't like about rubbers is it made him
go a long, long time." The fear of leakage, slippage, and even breakage
also can make sex with condoms unappealing. As Donna said,

I was thinking the whole time he was using them was that that thing was going to
burst, 'cause his penis was very large, and that's all I kept thinking about. That
that thing would burst. And I couldn't really get into the thing thinking that
rubber is gonna burst.

Donna's fear "that that thing would burst" indicates that condom users
and non-users think about condoms differently. While condom-using

women feel safer with condoms, non-users like Donna may feel safer — and more sexually fulfilled — without. Further, condom users are able to engage in self-protection without self-denigration. This is because they either cast condom use as a form of birth control, which says nothing about partners' fidelity, or they do not assume that if partner unfaithfulness does exist that it will detract from their own esteem or status. In such cases, condom-use may add to women's self-esteem as Alternative Wisdom Narratives and narratives about self-respect or, as focus group participants called it, "self-love" are put into play.

If Shelly's case is typical, it may be that the less a woman depends on her man for status and self-esteem, the more likely she will be to use condoms for HIV-transmission prevention. In the following section, some of the concrete structural factors that seem to differentiate users from non-users are identified and described.

Extraconjugal Factors

Affiliative Needs and Social Support

In the first phase of the study, participants talked about their desires for conjugal closeness and many described how these were accommodated or met through unsafe sex. They also reported keeping to themselves and maintaining few friends. That is, many women reported having small or weak extraconjugal support systems. So in the second phase of the research, I explored the possibility that women with lower levels of extraconjugal support might depend more on their conjugal partners to meet their emotional and social needs and so might experience a more intense need to idealize and justify their relationships and to deny the possibility of conjugal problems, as through unsafe sex. Similar patterns, albeit with outcome measures other than unsafe sex, have been documented for other groups of people.

Couvade, where a father-to-be experiences symptoms of the pregnancy, is a practice found in some cultures that cast pregnancy as a joint conjugal endeavor. Accordingly, pregnant women's partners exhibit pregnancy-related symptoms. In a study of couvade in Colombia, Carole Browner (1983) found that the number and severity of pregnancy-related symptoms women reported for their men were inversely correlated with the strength of the women's social networks. Women who felt more isolated tended to focus on the strength of their conjugal bond and on the way that couvade symptoms in their partners expressed this. Elizabeth Bott's work on conjugal relations and social networks in urban London (1957) documents the same kinds of correspondences between extraconjugal support and conjugal style (although variables such as shared recreational activities and joint decision-making rather than couvade symptoms were examined).

It is well known that the level of support offered by an individual's social circle influences health behaviors. As Orth-Gomer and Unden (1987) note in their review of the literature on measures of social support, "The frequency of social contacts, the number of available persons and the amount of social activities seem to have a substantial effect on health and survival" (83; also see Medalie et al. 1981; Schmidt 1978; Turner et al. 1989, 291–93). A correlation may exist between unsafe sex and weak extraconjugal social support just as a correlation existed between couvade symptom reports and social isolation.[10] To facilitate testing the hypothesis that unsafe sex and extraconjugal support are linked, William Dressler's definition of social support as "the perceived availability of help or assistance from other persons during times of felt need" and his definition of a "social support system" as "a subset of an individual's ego-centered social network" (1991, 19) were followed as the second-phase questionnaire and interview were developed.

The questionnaire asked women to indicate on a six-part Likert-type scale ranging from "never" to "always" how happy they were with their interactions with friends and relations, and whether or not they felt secure and supported.[11] A pattern suggesting that low levels of social support are associated with condomlessness emerged from pilot questionnaire data. Some of the questions were refined for the final version of the questionnaire. The frequencies reported below reflect the views of the participants who completed the final version.

Equal numbers of condom users and non-users had friends or relations that they relaxed with, and equal numbers had friends or relations on whom they could count for financial assistance when they needed it. Women also felt lonely with similar frequency or infrequency whether or not they used condoms. But while only one of the ten condom-using women felt that she generally (i.e., "always" or "very often") had "no one to turn to for help," six (17.6%) of the thirty-four non-users felt this way. And while five (50%) of the ten users reported that they could frequently (i.e., "always" or "very often") rely on friends and relatives for advice, only eleven (32.4%) of the non-users did so.

Social network data were also gathered from clinic interviewees. As Table 4 shows, only one of the six interviewees who used condoms during their last sexual encounters with their primary partners[12] considered her partner to be among her two closest social companions, while exactly half of the eighteen non-users did so. Users' lists of their two closest social companions contained slightly more relatives than the lists of non-users did, and they also contained slightly more women. Further, while only one of the six users (16.7%) talked about having a jealous partner, twelve

TABLE 4. Conjugal Patterns, Partner Jealousy, and Condom Use Among Clinic Interviewees

Partner is:	Users (N=6)	Non-users (N=18)
A close companion	1	9
Not a close companion	5	9
Jealous	1	12
Not jealous	5	6

(66.6%) or two in three non-users had jealous partners (a total of thirteen women or 52% deemed their partners jealous men). The interview data suggests that women with jealous partners are more dependent on their men for emotional and social resources and that their social circles are kept small by and for their men. This may lead them to be more likely to list their partners as close social companions.

Interviewee testimony informs the hypothesis that a link exists between conjugal styles, extraconjugal support systems, and AIDS-risk denial. The small size of the sample notwithstanding, the testimony suggests that there may be significant differences in the ways that users and non-users relate to their conjugal partners, and in the quality as well as the quantity of their extraconjugal social relations.

Roberta explained that her partner is jealous, saying he's "nosy, yes, [like] 'Who's that on the phone?' . . . If a guy calls me up, he just sits there right in my face while I'm talking to the guy on the phone, trying to figure out what the guy is saying." Rose had a similar problem:

I would let the phone ring and just let him pick it up so he won't think it was [a man], you know. I even went as far as buying a phone where he can hear our conversations. I just do that 'cause when I be talking, I'll just be saying "yeah, yeah, OK, uh-huh," and he'll be thinking I'm talking to a [man]. So I bought a speaker phone where he could hear the conversations. Then it got so bad — every time I'm not at home and the phone would ring he would say, "Is your boyfriend calling here and hanging up?" So I bought an answering machine so he could screen the calls.

Earlier, Rose had said of her partner, "He's always paranoid, you know. He is not one of those physical jealous men; it's more like verbal, you know." Rose gets tired of her partner's jealous ways, but she understands them. She explained that his past relationships and his upbringing might have led him to feel paranoid about female fidelity:

I think it's something that happened to him like in the past with his other women and stuff. I told him I thought that he [had] real mental problems. I really thought that he needed psycho [i.e., psychological help]. But he said when he was a little boy his mother told him. So I guess he always lived like that [i.e., jealously], 'cause his mother told him that he could never keep a woman. So I think his way—his mother had a lot of men, 'cause I know all his brothers and sisters got different fathers. You see what I'm saying? [He's used to thinking] that's the way women are.

Clarissa, who keeps very few friends, describes her situation: "All my friends were male and so I had to leave them all alone, and then the one [female] friend that I had, he can't stand her 'cause she's not married." Jealous partners like Clarissa's do not trust their women around other men, and they do not like them to socialize with single girlfriends. As Marvelle explains, "He figures they have an influence on me." Betsy said the same thing: "He thinks that they're going to introduce me to a guy."

Minutes earlier in the interview Betsy, who likes to spend time by herself playing solitaire, watching television, or reading books ("like Stephen King"), had said,

He's jealous. He wants me to stay in all the time. Don't even want me to see my mom. If I'm over to my mom's house, he's always thinks that me and my sisters have a guy over there for—everywhere I go he thinks that it's because a guy is there for me or I'm gonna have an affair.

She continued, "I guess because of the way he used to mess around, that's why he thinks that I'm going to do it." Penny also suspected that her partner's sexual patterns influenced his desire to keep a close watch on her. But in addition to fueling his suspicions, Penny also thought that her partner's affairs (which were ongoing and not just in the past, as for Betsy's man) might have caused him to fear that she would hear about his exploits if she patronized their neighborhood bar: "I don't know if he was [afraid of me seeing] the people that was down there, or—if he had somebody that he was dating down there, I don't know." (Penny was not on good terms with her partner, who, as mentioned previously, drank and neglected her and their baby.)

Adrienne's boyfriend was in jail, but even so he did not want her enjoying herself at bars. "He said that I wasn't supposed to be out partying when he was locked up," she told me, adding "He's selfish." Later Adrienne talked about an argument she had with her partner over having to curtail her outings with friends: "He's saying my friends was taking me to a new guy. I told him, 'I don't need nobody to take me to meet no new guy. I can meet a guy on my own if I wanted a new guy.' "

Sarah also focused on her partner's suspicions when discussing his jealousy. She explained, "When the relationship first started off, I had a lot of man friends. [My partner] thought it was more of a sexual thing [with them]. I told him it wasn't like that: they was just friends." But Sarah had to leave them behind in order to keep her partner happy. Beside men, her partner also does not like Sarah to spend time with people he does not know. When asked why, she said, "I asked him that, and he said " 'Cause I don't know [them and] ain't no telling what you all be up to.' " Marvelle's partner tells her, " 'You don't go out. Only whores go out.' " Peg's partner is "constantly, he's so jealous that I think he should go — like if I'm riding in the car, if I look this way in the car [she moves her head as if looking out of a car window], he goes 'Oh, you're looking there, why don't you just go on and get in the other car with the nigger-man?' He's extremely jealous."

Jealousy also is expressed in male opinions about their partners' attire and overall appearance. Sarah told me, "He doesn't like me wearing tight clothes; he really don't like it . . . He says, 'Don't you ever wear that around there ever again.' " She added, "I don't like that."[13] Similarly, Dee's beau does not want her wearing makeup ("sometimes he'd take his handkerchief and smear my makeup on my face when we're driving so I have to take it off") or tight skirts. She said he thinks that "everybody wants to look at my butt. [He says,] 'I don't want anybody thinking about [your] butt but [me]. Anytime I go to a party, [he says], 'You don't wear that short dress 'cause it's showing your butt too much." Donna said of her partner:

He's jealous. Because sometimes from the remarks he makes — like [when] we go to the grocery store or something and he's like, "I bet you be in here flirting with men like how we met," and I was like, "Oh please!" When I first do my hair or something, he'll say, "Maybe I should go with you." Or I'll have on a dress and heels and he'll be like, "Oh you look too good to go somewhere by yourself." And he tries to play about it, but he's kind of serious. I know he's serious.

Male control over female social circles is not only driven by men's fears that their women will commit adultery or leave them. Men's desires to spend time with their partners can lead them to act jealously. As many couples do not live together, time alone can be a rarity. "Sometimes he has a fit, like this Friday," said Dee, explaining that her partner told her " 'You're going to just stay here with just me, that's just it.' " He's posses-sive, she said, because he "just wants that private night." Moreover, as Nicole explained, male reputation concerns also play a role:

[To socialize with] my mother, then that's OK. But like if I was to stay here [and socialize with] my friend Tom, [my partner] would be like "No." No, men are out; that's just totally no way. It's not because — I don't think [my partner gets] scared. It's just that he's the kind of guy that worries about what people think of him, so if somebody was to see me and Tom, you know, and come and tell [my partner], "Well I've seen [Nicole] with Tom," you know, it's "Oh God!"

Men's jealousy limits women's social circles, forcing women to be more emotionally and socially dependent on their primary partners. Further, as a few of the interviews revealed, men's jealousy can sometimes find expression in more extreme forms of controlling behavior, like verbal and physical abuse. Women with few outside sources of support — without a sense of "home" extraconjugally — can find themselves trapped, as Peg explained:

> [My partner] was real jealous and he got to be controlling and abusive, physically abusive towards me, but I still tried to hang in there because he had all the qualities that I wanted at that time — that I thought that I wanted in a man. When he got abusive I would say [to myself], "What do you think?" and I sat and thought about it, I said, "Well, it was my fault. I should have just shut my mouth up." I was more or less yearning for those type of men and I loved those men and I was a dope. And I was basically trying to find a home. . . . Those kind of men they protect you and then it's like they know just when to romance you in the right way and just when to try to discipline, or put their control, like when they see you kinda getting on your own and getting away from them.

Peg's mention of protection is important: some women who have controlling partners see that control as beneficial (cf. Pivnick 1993). Winsome, for instance, who only recently quit using drugs, defended her boyfriend's insistence on guarding her: "In a way I like it 'cause he takes care of me." She knows that he does not want her to slide back into using drugs, and she says that some may think of him as "being mean, but it's only because he loves me." Earlier, when we talked about why she loved her partner, she said, "He's a good man. He never gave up on me [when I was using]."

Well-meaning or not, jealous men who, in Peg's words, "put their control" seek to suppress women's independence. "Getting on your own and getting away from them" might involve employment, which Winsome's boyfriend, like Peg's, would not allow. "Getting on your own" always involves extraconjugal contacts, which threaten jealous men because they believe that such contacts promote over-independence in women and possible adulterous liaisons. Clinic focus group participant Betty explained that some men purposefully promote women's dependence:

> If [a woman has] got a lot of friends and a lot of family to talk to and stuff, she's not so dependent on that man. [Women get dependent on a man if] he don't want her to have outside friends. Or family here — he don't want no family participating. If the family tells her the sky blue, he say it's green. The sky blue, but [what he says is what she] goes by. He don't want her to listen to her family and friends.

Contradicting the monogamy ideal and undermining the Monogamy Narrative is extremely threatening in this kind of situation, so women with jealous or controlling partners are perhaps the most likely to be nonusers of condoms. Indeed, as noted, only one (16.7%, N = 6) condom using interviewee portrayed her partner as jealous, while, twelve (66.6%, N = 18) non-using interviewees did so.

Women and Friendship

Earlier, I mentioned that participants in the first phase of the study reported keeping to themselves and maintaining few friends. Clinic interviews indicate that this is due in part to partner jealousy. Dee said of a female friend that her partner would rather she not see, "He thinks I spend too much time with her. If I don't fix [fresh] dinner, [he says,] 'Why are you giving me that old grub?' [I say,] 'I had to go take her out somewhere,' [and he says,] 'You don't do that for me.' "

But isolation is not solely due to men's wishes. Many interviewees expressed little interest of their own in socializing. Michelle's declarations, "I don't keep a lot of friends," "I'm just quiet," and "I'm more like a private person," Betsy's statement, "I can be social but I don't like to, not too much," Sarah's pronouncement, "I don't have too many women friends; I don't have too many friends, period," and Donna's blunt statement, "I don't have any friends," were typical of many interviewees.

Mary said, "I used to have friends but I didn't understand life, the value of life. No, I don't have any friends [now.]" Friends keep people from taking the righteous, sober path, she said, adding, "I'm being honest, honey. I don't know how anybody else sees it, but I'm telling you exactly how I feel."

Peg pointed to the responsibilities that motherhood brings rather than focusing on the trouble that friends can involve, explaining, "I don't hang out or anything. I'm at home. I'm playing with my kids . . . I ain't got no more time for nothing else. Kids keep you busy, you know." A few minutes later, she said, "I don't have people coming in and out of my doors. [My partner] loves it 'cause it's secluded like that. It's basically just me and him." Rose, who similarly said, "My main way is to be homebound," stated simply, "My partner is my best friend."

Five of the twenty-five clinic interviewees (20%) counted their partners as their best friends; five more (20%) counted them as their second closest companions (regarding the lack of condom use among these women, see Table 4, in the preceding section). Mary instructed me, "You don't need people [i.e., friends]. The only person you need is that man for you and that's enough. If you can understand him and yourself, you don't need to be around other people." "He's my best friend. I can say that, 'cause I can tell him anything, you know," said Sarah.

The discontinuity between condom use and considering lovers as close friends was made clear in a focus group discussion in which one participant called the group's attention to the optimistic bias, asking, "How many of us in here are using condoms with our man?" Someone quickly declared in response (and in defense), "Our mates are our friends."

Twelve clinic interviewees (48%) found keeping female friends particularly dangerous. This was not only because their partners did not like them to do so, but also because, as the women explained, so-called friends often do not have one's best interests in mind. As Mary said, "People can get you in a lot of trouble." So the narrowness of some women's social circles seems to be related not only to partner jealousy but also to their own selective preference for solitude. And women who preferred fewer friends were, like women with jealous partners and those with partners as close companions, less likely to be condom-users. Of the six condom-using women, only one saw keeping female friends as dangerous. Sometimes, women fear that their so-called friends will advertise their secrets to the world; other times, they fear that their so-called friends will try to steal their partners away (in this section, I use "friends" only in reference to females, or girlfriends, as did the interviewees). As Roberta explained, "Friends could take your boyfriend or husband away from you. They can slander your name, you know—things you tell them in confidence they can tell someone else."

Rose said,

I don't really want a best friend. I can't even say I have a best friend, no, no. 'Cause your best friend—you could tell a best friend anything and I don't have one of those. My partner is my best friend . . . I never trust women . . . It would be [him]. I have a cousin—she's pretty close. I mean, I can talk to her and not worry about it going anywhere . . . I can trust her with anything[14]

Twenty-three-year-old Shelly said, "I'm very picky about who I take on as friends and talk with as friends, and I feel confidence in them, you know. You have to say things to see if they ain't gonna break [that confidence] and tell another [person your secrets]."

In addition to breaking confidences by spreading one's secrets, so-called friends can break confidences by "trying to take your boyfriend," as Betsy bluntly pointed out. Nicole said, "I just worry about that if my girl was to try and talk to my man and my man was to tell me—you know I'm not jealous, I'm hurt." Nicole assumed and so implied, by saying that her man would tell her about her girlfriend's advances, that he would have rebuffed them. Even so, like most of the interviewees Nicole would, in another context, agree with Shelly's statement, "A man's never committed totally. He's gonna mess around." Many interviewees—or at least many of those who did not use condoms—felt that since so-called friends are quite likely to take advantage of one's man's "natural" propensity to "mess around," then so-called friends are better avoided.

Numerous interviewees described female friends as "back-stabbers" in explaining their preferences for solitude. Twenty-two-year-old Penny said that she did not keep many friends because "I don't trust them, get in a lot of trouble. 'Cause in my younger years I was stabbed in the back a lot." In discussing her job as a nurse's aide in a home for the aged, Nicole said,

It's just like a total competition always with women, you know. It really is. [Women are] way more competitive [than men . . .]. It's just always somebody trying to back-stab you, and it's always somebody trying to get in your mix and tell every-body about, you know, on the next shift or something.

Clarissa said, "They want to try to kill you, you know, stab [you in the back.] I'm very selective." "They are back-stabbers," declared Bernice, who continued, "Can't trust them. You can never say you have a best friend, because there ain't—they always change into something differ-ent. You thought you could trust them but you couldn't. You always helped them out and then [they turn on you]."

The Condom Conundrum

In addition to suggesting that many women are active players in sexual decisions and that financial coercion plays only a minor role in driving unsafe sex, study findings suggest that there is a positive correlation be-tween unsafe sex and emotional and social dependence on men. Impov-erished inner-city women idealize monogamy and hope for loyal conju-gal partners. Much of their relationship-related talk describes a dream of fidelity, puts forth a claim of having achieved it, or supports a belief in its reality. Because condoms are associated with infidelity and deceptive behavior, using them implies that partners do not truly care for one another. Admitting to this in regard to one's own relationship is emo-tionally painful and shaming. Condom use undermines the Monogamy (and Wisdom) Narratives that women are encouraged to and need to tell; therefore, it is avoided.

Women who are less dependent on men for self-esteem and support—women who have strong extraconjugal networks that they feel good about—are less likely to forgo condoms. But women with small social networks or weak extraconjugal ties may tend to focus on their con-jugal relationships more than other women do, and so may tend to en-gage in more of the wishful thinking about monogamy that denial and unsafe sex entail. The less convinced women are that friends and relatives will take care of them, the more likely they are to have unsafe sex—the more likely they are to engage in wishful thinking and denial during the emotionally charged period of lovemaking. This may be exacerbated in some cases by joblessness, as some women without jobs may be forced to rely more on relationships with men for self-esteem than on their own accomplishments.

Women who agree with and aspire to fulfill mainstream relationship ideals put themselves in danger by practicing unsafe sex. Supporting one's denial of the possibility of a partner's infidelity by having unsafe sex is an adaptive, psychosocially beneficial practice in the short run. But this strategy can have deadly long-term costs — especially when invoked in the context of poverty and sexism.

Substandard health care, the frequency of intravenous drug use and untreated venereal infection (see Ward 1993a), the negative effects of economic oppression on gender relations, and the high prevalence of HIV in impoverished inner-city environments mean that poor urban women who have unsafe sex are at a higher risk for HIV infection than their better-off peers. The next chapter explores HIV testing for women at risk. It considers the pros and cons of testing, focusing on women's attitudes toward and beliefs about testing, and on their self-reported testing practices.

*   *   *

Much of the material in this chapter was adapted from "Inner-City Women and AIDS: The Psycho-Social Benefits of Unsafe Sex," *Culture, Medicine, and Psychiatry* 17 (4) (1993): 455–485.

Notes

1. Here, I should note that the effective size of one's social network depends less on the sheer number of individuals that it contains than on the perceived support that those individuals (or a subset thereof) can provide in times of need (cf. Dressler 1991). Sometimes women with numerically large networks feel undersupported because they perceive the people in their networks as meddlesome and as harboring ill will toward them.

2. This line of questioning was not pursued in the clinic interviews.

3. 9 percent of white men and 13 percent of Black men said that they used condoms "always."

4. Note that the data described (Catania et al. 1993) were collected in 1989 and 1990; more recent data would probably indicate higher frequencies of consistent use on all fronts.

5. See note 6, Chapter 6.

6. Participants say that women often cheat, too, but are more likely than men to deny it. According to Blumstein and Schwartz (1983, as cited in Turner et al. 1989, 110–11), 21 percent of married and 30 percent of cohabiting women have extraconjugal sex. However, because Blumstein and Schwartz's sample was only 5

percent African American, and because African American women appear to have more conservative sexual repertoires and fewer partners than white women (e.g., Worth 1990; Wyatt 1988, as cited in Turner et al. 1989, 112), a downward adjustment may be needed. At any rate, participants say that women who cheat are even more worried and in deeper denial about their partners' infidelities, because they project their own desires and behaviors onto their men.

7. Both an initial response and a secondary one were recorded for the sighting scenario. The data described here reflect the total content of each woman's answer.

8. The link between women's self-empowerment and insistence on condom use seen here fits with Ward's finding that family planning programs only work when contraceptive practice is perceived as empowering (1991).

9. See note 6.

10. I thank Jill Korbin for this suggestion.

11. Interestingly, most of the women who failed to provide information were not condom-users, and the questions that they did provide answers for showed that they were generally under-supported.

12. A seventh interviewee had used a condom during her last sexual encounter but as this was with an outside partner she is excluded from the analyses in this section.

13. Sarah also told me, "I'm gonna wear it anyway," asserting her independence. Indeed, she wore shorts to the interview. Other women with jealous, watchful men were not as self-determined as Sarah; they upheld the standards that their men set for them.

14. Women often think of well-liked female kin as friends. Many said that their mothers were their best friends.

Chapter 8
HIV Testing and Wishful Thinking

Condomless sex supports the Monogamy Narratives women tell about themselves and their relationships. A positive HIV test leads a woman to replace this narrative with another: as Martha Ward (1993b) shows, many HIV-positive women tell of broken trust and partners that must not have really loved them. I call this narrative the "Betrayal Narrative."[1]

Even prior to and without positive diagnoses, women fear betrayal. A woman may believe in her own wisdom and skill in choosing safe partners, and she may trust her man when he says that he is faithfully monogamous. But, for reasons connected to risk perception (see Chapter 3), probing questions asked in the context of actual HIV testing will probably reveal that she also believes that if anything will lead to a positive test it will be her partner's misbehavior and his lack of concern for her well-being — not her own high-risk action. The frequency of male betrayal (abandonment, abuse, etc.) helps explain the prominence of the theme and the assumption. Importantly, the extrapunitive thinking underlying this assumption releases women from responsibility for the possible consequences of what are actually their own unsafe practices (e.g., having condomless sex with a non-monogamous partner).

Positive tests lead to Betrayal Narratives, which are hindsighted depositions of a partner's disloyalty and deceit. But what leads to testing in the first place if women do not see themselves at risk? What do women think and feel about HIV tests and the testing process? These are the questions that this chapter addresses.

Testing Recommendations

Because of the increasing frequency of HIV infection among impoverished urban Blacks and because HIV can be passed on in pregnancy, inner-city public health care workers often urge pregnant clients and those who have histories of high-risk behaviors (such as intravenous drug use or condomless sex) to consider having their blood tested for HIV antibodies. Sometimes HIV-testing policy decisions related to women stem from concern about pediatric AIDS, suggesting that women's health is important only insofar as women can serve as HIV carriers. Other times, policy makers see women's health as being important in and of itself; in this case, pregnancy simply affords clinicians the opportunity to test women for HIV, as expectant women generally use clinic services much more frequently than women who are not (and who have not recently been) pregnant.

The CDC and most public health officials recommend that preconception and prenatal HIV testing routinely be offered to women considered to have a high risk[2] for HIV infection. Officials advise that pre- and post-test counseling accompany all tests because of the possible psychological ramifications of seropositivity and also because counselors can educate clients about prevention and, when necessary, about treatment (Coates et al. 1988; Kurth and Hutchison 1989; Lindsay et al. 1990, 1989; regarding the psychological ramifications of testing positive, see Chapter 4). Most research on HIV tests for women focuses on the measurable costs and benefits of testing for prevention and treatment efforts (e.g., Pappaioanou et al. 1990 or the papers just cited) or it concerns ethical matters, such as confidentiality and permissions (e.g., Boyd 1990). Determinants of testing, which this chapter deals with, have received little attention (an exception is Mantell et al. 1992).

Many caregivers, clients, and researchers have their doubts about testing. For example, many researchers question HIV-screening guidelines. Lindsay et al. (1989) found that testing on the basis of self-reported risk factors was extremely inefficient, as testing only those inner-city minority women who perceive themselves as being at risk for HIV infection would omit from testing and so conceal as much as 70 percent of all seropositive cases. Similarly, using data from a San Francisco STD clinic, Onorato et al. (1994) show that "voluntary testing detected only 44 percent of the HIV-infected STD clients and that voluntary testing underestimated the prevalence of HIV among clinic attendees by 35 percent" (206).

Screening criteria issues notwithstanding, many testing advocates celebrate the health-enhancing benefits of early intervention. But treatment is not often readily available for HIV-positive individuals in impoverished inner-city settings, where even basic health care can be difficult to come by (Lazarus 1990; Ward 1993a; see also Dalton 1989; Thomas and Quinn 1991; and Quimby 1992 regarding racism and health care). Information concerning how to reduce one's risk for HIV infection through safer sex (and, for IDUs, through the use of household bleach in syringes and needles) is generally the most substantive aid that public health care workers who serve poor urban populations can offer.

Simply participating in conjoined HIV testing and counseling has been associated with subsequent risk reduction among homosexual men and IDUs in some studies; the highest rates of risk reduction are generally reported by those participants who test positive (Coates et al. 1988; Turner et al. 1989, 281). But other studies done with these populations find no correlations (e.g. Doll et al. 1990; Landis et al. 1992) and still others indicate that significant amounts of behavioral backsliding occur (see Miller et al. 1990; Stall et al. 1990). In any case, few studies that examine the ways that HIV testing and counseling are related to reduced risk-taking focus on women—excepting those women who are pregnant. Even for this group few data exist, as studies of pregnant women who have been tested usually focus on their decisions regarding pregnancy termination (e.g., Arras 1990, Levine and Dubler 1990, Pivnick et al. 1991). The issues surrounding the view of women as only disease vectors notwithstanding (Carovano 1991; see also Herdt and Boxer 1991), pregnancy does seem to motivate lowered AIDS risk taking (Mays and Cochran 1988; Tunstall et al. 1991). But it does not necessarily motivate testing.

As I explained in Chapter 2, while pregnant women considering testing are generally concerned about passing HIV on to their babies-to-be (Mays and Cochran 1988; Tunstall et al. 1991; Ward 1993a; regarding altruism, see also Turner et al. 1989, 279), few pregnant inner-city women actually get tested for HIV before their pregnancies are well underway (Lindsay et al. 1990; regarding barriers to prenatal care, see Lazarus 1990). Tested or not, an infected woman's chances of giving birth to a healthy, AIDS-free child are relatively high: only about one-fourth of all babies born to HIV-positive mothers will develop AIDS. In light of the other odds and obstacles that inner-city women regularly face, this gamble can seem minimal (Campbell 1990; Carovano 1991; Catania et al. 1990; Levine and Dubler 1990; see also Chapter 9). Besides, legal restrictions, social and cultural pressures, financial hardships, and some clinicians' misgivings about exposing themselves to HIV can make getting abortions very difficult for seropositive inner-city women who would chose to do so.

The factors I have mentioned limit the value that many women see in HIV testing for the prevention of perinatal or mother-child transmission. The recent finding that therapy with the drug AZT (azidothymidine) significantly reduces a baby's chance of infection (CDC 1994b) may change this—if AZT is made available to poor inner-city women.[3] In any case, the value women place on testing in other situations and with other goals in mind has remained an open question.

Testing Barriers: Target Group Views

When HIV testing is offered in a clinic, clients weigh many factors. The scant research focusing on the determinants of women's voluntary uptake of testing generally involves easily quantifiable variables like education, race or ethnicity, income, religion, acquaintance with persons who have already been tested, and so forth (e.g., Mantell et al. 1992). The relevant dimensions of broadly defined variables such as these cannot be identified without considering clients' experiences and attitudes directly and in detail, as this research does, providing for a richer understanding of test-related behavior (cf. Lang 1991). The following brief review of the health concerns of the disenfranchised (see also Chapter 3) and of some of the findings from the first phase of the research provides a context within which to view the test-determinant data from the second phase.

The experience of racism and the legacy of the negative encounters that Blacks have had with the public health system, as well as the mistreatment that women and the poor have historically received from the biomedical sector (Corea 1992; Lazarus 1990), fuel the misgivings that many Black women have about health-care workers' motives and intents. Many inner-city women recognize the questionable quality of the health care that they will receive if seropositive, and they recognize the health-care delivery system challenges that they will face (Corea 1992; Ward 1993a; cf. Lazarus 1990).

The problematic nature of prevention further undermines women's desire for testing. Inner-city women often feel, sometimes fatalistically, that there is little they can do to reduce their chances of infection (Dorfman et al. 1992). Although, as studies show, AIDS knowledge levels among Black women generally are high (e.g., Flaskerud and Rush 1989; Hardy and Biddlecom 1991; Harrison et al. 1991; Jemmott and Jemmott 1991; Johnson 1993), many still fear that AIDS can be spread through casual contact or through doorknobs and public toilets because "you never know" (Flaskerud and Rush 1989, 212; see also Hardy and Biddlecom 1991; Schoenborn et al. 1994). Indeed, as I noted in Chapter 3, participants in the focus groups held during the first phase of the research expressed such concerns during discussions in which modes of transmission were correctly identified and adeptly discussed. They also voiced doubts about the prophylactic value of condoms — doubts they backed up with references to current scientific disagreements, media reports about condom leakage and breakage, propaganda promoted by groups like the Nation of Islam (cf. Thomas and Quinn 1991), and stories about personal experiences of condom failure. Moreover, focus group participants pointed out that unprotected sex is just one of many ways to "catch

AIDS," which can be transmitted in an emergency blood transfusion or by a vindictive HIV-positive individual. They also noted that the risk of AIDS is itself but one more risk among a multitude of others that they face daily (cf. Catania et al. 1990; Mays and Cochran 1988; Worth 1989).

Risk (Mis)Perception

As shown in Chapters 3 and 7, the concept of perceived susceptibility has not proved too useful for safer-sex interventions, mostly because of the problems people have personalizing information about AIDS risks. When partners are considered faithful, women do not see themselves at risk for AIDS. It follows that the concept of perceived risk also would have little use in interventions involving testing, as women convinced of their partners' loyalty will see no logical reason to be tested for HIV. Indeed, because it might undermine their dreams of monogamy (and cost them their status and self-esteem), HIV testing based on a notion of personal risk should be, for these women, near to impossible.

I tested this premise by examining the beliefs and motivations of a sample of women that included HIV test-takers and seeking to isolate the factors associated with positive decisions to be tested. Guided by the assumption that behavior is driven by cultural logic, or reason as influenced by cultural context, and by emotion's effects on perceived susceptibility, I attempted to identify dimensions of the test-related decision-making process that could be employed in interventions designed to increase testing rates among M&I clients.

Results

Tested or Not?

As Table 5 shows, over two-thirds (68.4%, n = 13) of the 19 surveyed first-phase focus group women claimed to have had an HIV test. But when testing came up in discussion, most said that the tests were simply given to them, rather than requested by them; they also said that clinicians routinely check for HIV when drawing blood for other purposes.

In order to ascertain the likelihood that those women who thought they had been tested actually had been, they were asked if they talked about the experience with a clinician before or after the supposed test. While Ohio law requires pre- and post-test counseling and verbal or written consent (the type of consent required depends on whether the test is wholly anonymous or merely confidential), only three (23.1%) of the thirteen women who claimed to have been tested remembered signing papers or having been counseled in any way.

TABLE 5. HIV Test Status and Counseling Memories Among Focus Group
Participants and Questionnaire Respondents

	Focus group participants	Questionnaire respondents
Already tested	13 (68.4%, N = 19)	37 (41.1%, N = 90)
Recall pre-test counseling	n.a.	27 (79.4%, N = 34)*
Recall post-test counseling	n.a.	25 (75.6%, N = 33)*
Recall any counseling	3 (23.1%, N = 13)	n.a.

*While 37 women were tested, data were missing for 3 and 4 respectively.

In light of this finding, the clinic questionnaire included a question about memories of testing (see Table 5). Thirty-seven (41.1%) of the ninety questionnaire respondents reported having taken HIV tests; thirty- four and thirty-three provided information about pre- and post-test counseling, respectively. Twenty-seven (79.4%, N = 34) women received pre-test counseling; twenty-five (75.6%, N = 33) received post-test counseling.

The frequencies calculated for the clinic women were much higher than the figure calculated for focus group women (23.1%). This is heartening; I think it reflects the emphasis that M&I clinicians have been directed to place on AIDS education and on properly carried out HIV testing. Still, in at least one in five cases in the clinic, either no counseling at all occurred, or many women who think that they have been tested are mistaken.

Women's Preferences: To Test or Not to Test?

I mentioned that thirty-seven (41.1%) of the questionnaire respondents claimed to have had an HIV test. As Table 6 shows, sixteen (17.8%) more desired to be tested but had not yet been. Grouped together, these fifty-three pro-testing women make up almost three-fifths (58.9%) of the questionnaire respondents (regarding those with no desire to be tested, see Appendix B6). As Table 6 shows, a slightly larger total proportion of the eighteen first-phase interviewees (72.2%) wanted to be or had been tested: nine (50%) claimed to have been tested and four (22.2%) desired HIV tests (second-phase interviewees were not asked about testing; sufficient testing data had been collected and other avenues of questioning needed to be pursued).

Test-takers and would-be test-takers saw the HIV test primarily as a standard health evaluation procedure; this was their most common explanation for getting tested (see Table 6). The likelihood of invoking the idea of the test's routine nature varied according to whether the test had

TABLE 6. Test Status and Perceptions of Testing as Routine Among Questionnaire Respondents and First-Phase Interviewees

	Questionnaire respondents	First-phase interviewees
Already tested	37 (41.1%, N=90)	9 (50%, N=18)
Believe HIV tests are routine	26 (70.3%, N=37)	5 (55.6%, N=9)
Desire to be tested	16 (17.8%, N=90)	4 (22.2%, N=18)
Believe HIV tests are routine	10 (62.5%, N=16)	4 (100%, N=4)
Have been or desire to be tested: total	53 (58.9%, N=90)	13 (72.2%, N=18)
Believe HIV tests are routine	36 (67.9%, N=53)	9 (69.2%, N=13)

already been taken or was desired. But while for interviewees this likelihood was higher among those who desired the test than among those who had already taken it, for questionnaire respondents, the opposite was found. Only five (55.6%) of the nine interviewed women who said they had been tested explained testing as normal, while all four interviewees who desired the test talked of it as routine. Inversely, twenty-six (70.3%) of the thirty-seven questionnaire respondents who claimed to have been tested talked about the test's routine nature, while only ten (62.5%) of the sixteen who desired HIV tests cast HIV testing as a standard procedure.

Partners' Practices, Women's Risks

Tested or not, few of the women who did mention their risks for AIDS talked about being at risk as if this was something they were personally responsible for. Over half the 13 focus group women surveyed who had been or wanted to be tested voiced concerns about their partners' behaviors (regarding the importance of context in interpreting such reported concerns, see below). Fewer of the 53 questionnaire respondents who had been or who wanted to be tested (23.1%, n = 12)[4] expressed any indication that their conjugal relations might be risky (see Appendix B6). Admittedly, this might have been because a questionnaire format leaves no room for the kind of self-reflective discussion that focus groups can draw from women.

The women who did report a sense of risk were far more likely to charge their partners than themselves with responsibility for the risk. None of the nineteen surveyed focus group women said that they themselves were taking risks, and only one of the eighteen first-phase interviewees[5] thought that her own sexual behavior put her at risk (she had two sex partners).[6] Similarly, only one questionnaire respondent (N = 90) said that she was taking risks (she had had sex without condoms).

Discussion

Fidelity

In their discourse, many women suggested that new partners should get checked for HIV together. But only a few examples of this happening can be found in the study data. One focus group participant, who had already been tested herself, said,

[My partner and I] discussed AIDS, but when we came to that [i.e., sex], he was like, "Rubber? I haven't ever used a rubber." I told him to go get an AIDS test. So he went like a stupid, he went, and waited, and when it came back we thought about it. I showed him mine . . . So that's why I had sex with him without a rubber.

The gender-role expectation-related implications of the statement that "he went like a stupid" notwithstanding, the woman took the negative results as a green light for unsafe sex. Clinic-interviewee Donna and her boyfriend did the same. Donna wanted to use condoms with her partner when they first met. However, she said,

He was so against rubbers that he went to the Free Clinic and got a blood test. I told him, "I don't have AIDS," because I just had my tubes tied, and my AIDS test was A-OK. I told him, "I don't have it." So he said he hadn't done anything with nobody for nine months. I said, "Well, just think, that person you did something with nine months ago could have had AIDS." So he went to the Free Clinic. . . . I said, "How can you tell me you don't have anything when you don't know yourself? You go take that blood test and then we'll both know." And right now, well, I know he's not messin' around with nobody.

These women's stories demonstrate one of the problematic ways in which serostatus information from a single HIV test can be made use of. That is, negative test results can be taken as permission to go ahead with unsafe sex because of the assumption that infection cannot happen after the date of the test. Also, negative results can help women to distance themselves mentally from the pandemic and they can support a woman's perception that she is in control of her life in relation to HIV-related risk and so need not use condoms (Kinsey 1994).

Beyond tests for new partners which, despite women's endorsement of the idea, seemed actually to happen rarely (perhaps largely because of the Wisdom Narrative's impact on women's calculations of risk in relation to new partners), women admitted that when fears of a long term partner's infidelity protrude into consciousness too often for comfort, they can check on his faithfulness by getting tested themselves. Participants said that "you never really know" about your partner, and that an HIV test is a way to check on a partner's supposed faithfulness. One surveyed focus group participant wrote, "I feel that [the HIV test] would let me know how my partner feels about my life." Another woman bluntly wrote, "My partner may be getting sex from someone else." An interviewee in the first phase said, "Some men lie. . . . I wonder what he's done since we last saw each other." These reasons reflect women's fear of (often unavoidable) betrayal.

Importantly, suspicion about a partner's practices was voiced only in relation to justifying the HIV test or as a general qualifier for statements confirming his faithfulness. For example, a woman would say that her man was completely trustworthy and then qualify this with a statement indicating that one can never really know what others are up to. This is a rhetorical ploy that will protect a woman's ego should she ever become convinced of her mate's infidelities. She can then say, "I knew it all along." Scientists also qualify their predictions: "The sun may not rise tomorrow, but we are reasonably sure that it will."

Test Uptake Figures

I relied on self-reports of testing in this research because clinic data were not available and also because the literature on HIV-related self-reports suggests that they are reliable. O'Campo et al. (1992) found that women's self-reports of HIV serostatus correlated almost perfectly with their medical records. McCusker et al. (1992) tested the validity of self-reported HIV-antibody test results, found it generally high, and so deemed self-reports appropriate in certain cases, as when laboratory confirmation is unavailable. In the end, what proved most important methodologically was that using self-reports led to a productive and innovative line of ethnographic inquiry regarding the test that otherwise might not have been investigated.

A relatively large proportion of the women who participated in this research claimed to have been tested for HIV. Among focus group participants, the proportion was almost seven in ten (68.4%); among questionnaire respondents it was more than two in five (41.1%). Maternity clinic based HIV testing is a relatively new practice and test delivery (and medical record access) protocols are still being developed. Studies show test uptake patterns to be complex and contingent on many factors, making broad comparisons between these data and data collected in other studies inappropriate as well as impracticable. Further, few global or national test acceptance statistics even exist against which I might compare the frequencies from this sample. U.S. HIV test uptake figures range from as low as 11 percent to as high as 99 percent, depending on who offers testing, how they offer it, and so forth (B. Caldwell and K. MacQueen, both of the CDC, 1993, personal communication). These facts must be borne in mind when reviewing the few available test uptake figures I present in the next few paragraphs.

According to results from the 1989 data set of the annual National Health Interview Survey (NHIS) of representative U.S. households (Anderson et al. 1992) — results based on self-reports[7] and which do not reflect the experiences of homeless, imprisoned, and hospital-bound people — over 20 percent (21.5%) of U.S. adults have been tested for HIV antibodies, mostly through blood donations, but also voluntarily or for military induction, immigration, or "other reasons." For Blacks, the statistic is just over 18 percent (18.3%).[8]

About 40 percent (41.5%) of persons "at increased risk"[9] in 1989 reported ever having been tested. Just less than half of these tests (19.9%) were voluntary. Among "at increased risk" Blacks in particular, 35 percent reported having been tested; about one-third of these tests (12.2%) were voluntary. Just as fewer Blacks than whites got tested, so too fewer women got tested than men: while about 45 percent of all "at increased risk" men got tested, only 37 percent of "at increased risk" women did so. And while slightly more than one-fifth (21.2%) of men "at increased risk" had voluntary tests, less than one-fifth (18.1%) of women "at increased risk" did so (Anderson et al. 1992).

Data from the 1992 NHIS (which is not confined to those "at increased risk") show that women are slightly more likely than men to report that they are not at risk for AIDS (67% as compared to 62%; Schoenborn et al. 1994). Risk perception data for gender groups according to ethnicity is available from the 1990 survey. Among Blacks, more women (75%) than men (70%) report that they are not at risk for AIDS (Hardy and Biddlecom 1991).[10] This helps to explain why in that year Black women were less likely than Black men to plan on testing in the future (12% and 17% respectively; p. 7).

The National Health Interview Survey was not designed solely with HIV testing in mind, and it certainly was not developed to target "increased risk" individuals. Another national survey (Berrios et al. 1993), which was, found that while 21 percent of U.S. adults in general had gotten tested, 23 percent of those living in cities deemed "high-risk" had done so (taken together, the "high-risk" cities contain about two-thirds of the nation's AIDS cases; they include Miami, New York, San Francisco, San Diego, etc.). One in four Blacks living in "high-risk" urban areas had been tested by 1990 to 1991, the years in which the survey was carried out.[11]

Counseling

As mentioned, a relatively large proportion of women participating in this study claimed to have taken the HIV test. However, despite the requirement for pre- and post-test counseling, in the case of the surveyed focus group members more than three in four could not recall having been counseled, and in the case of the questionnaire respondents the same was true for more than one in five women. Data regarding actual counseling frequencies in Cleveland's M&I clinics are not available. I was assured numerous times that M&I clinicians always counsel HIV testees; whether this is true I cannot say. I also do not know how many of the questionnaire respondent testees got tested through M&I and how many used other venues. So I will turn my attention to the focus group figures as I try to derive an estimate of the proportion of women who had not actually been tested for HIV antibodies although they said that they had been.

Data from two national studies of HIV screening in hospitals indicate that, despite recommendations and guidelines, counseling only takes place between 53 percent and 62 percent of the time (the former figure is from Henry et al. 1991, the latter from Freeman 1991).[12] If we use a slightly conservative average of these two figures (57%), we can speculatively estimate how many of the nineteen surveyed focus group participants actually were tested. For instance, we can guess that rather than being about 68 percent (n = 13; see Table 5), the actual test uptake frequency for the focus group sample was about 39 percent, because five or six of the women who reported having been tested but not counseled may not actually have been tested at all.[13] These participants might have lied about having been tested because they sought to please us, but because seeking testing can imply moral and social shortcomings (e.g., one's partner's or one's own promiscuity) and since reported condom use was extremely low (rather than inflated), it is safe to deem testing claims genuine — even if mistaken.

False Testing Claims?

Many focus group participants had erroneous beliefs about how HIV testing happens. Many assumed that any blood drawn by a clinician was checked for all pathogens, HIV included, even if they did not specifically request the HIV test. They were partially correct: various health care centers do send blood specimens to the CDC for use in a national prenatal, postnatal, and neonatal HIV seroprevalence survey. But every patient's blood is not sent. Further, officials cannot notify HIV carriers of their seropositivity because all personal identifying information is removed from seroprevalence survey samples (Pappaioanou et al. 1990).

Even participants who were not aware of seroprevalence survey testing frequently believed that blood drawn was automatically tested for HIV seropositivity and that, should HIV antibodies be found in their blood, they would be told. Some thought that testing was mandatory. Others thought that they were tested for HIV when in the hospital for surgical or other invasive procedures unrelated to AIDS, simply because that was the hospital routine.[14] Similarly, 17 percent of the women who participated in the 1992 National Health Interview Survey and who said that they had been tested for HIV said also that they were tested for hospitalization or a surgical procedure (Schoenborn et al. 1994).

While pondering the ramifications of the possibility that a large proportion of people wrongly think that they have been tested, I asked several white middle-class women about their experience with HIV tests; the same pattern of assumption emerged (cf. Lazarus 1990). For instance, it was assumed that a gynecological check-up would include an HIV test, particularly if a vaginal infection was present. A similar leap of faith also was made in an Institute of Medical Ethics (IME) Working Party paper written by Kenneth Boyd (1990). The paper describes a case in which a woman presumed that her doctor had given her an HIV test because, Boyd says, "The doctor knew, after all, that her ex-husband often worked abroad, and—well, all the reasons for the divorce" (173). Boyd and the Working Party take the accuracy of the woman's presumption for granted.

Abuses of power that result in unsolicited testing can occur and even well-intentioned clinicians—particularly overburdened public servants—sometimes cannot find time to carry out testing procedures properly (Corea 1992; cf. Lazarus 1990). A national survey of U.S. infectious disease teaching hospitals (Henry et al. 1991) found that consent for HIV tests was secured only 70 percent of the time. Ignorance about HIV-testing consent laws and guidelines, which I have encountered in caregivers as well as in clients, probably accounts for some of the tests given without permission. But participants generally attributed ideas about imposed testing to their own autonomous figuring (e.g., "I just figured it out myself") rather than to any specific external cues, like clinicians' statements (e.g., "I'm giving you an HIV test now"). This, and people's hesitancy to acknowledge their own AIDS risks, suggests that wishful thinking is at work when people assume themselves tested.

Clinicians—especially those in STD or prenatal clinics—must tell clients that blood drawn is not automatically tested for HIV, and they and all other clinicians must remain alert for false reports of previous testing. To check the accuracy of clients' impressions, they must ask direct questions about permissions, counseling experiences, and the manner in which results were received. Clinicians can then make educated guesses as to the validity of their clients' claims, and advise them accordingly. Not having received educational counseling previously, those who wrongly believe themselves to be certified free of HIV may also see themselves as risk-free, thinking perhaps that their sexual practices are "safer" or that since they did not contract HIV previously, they cannot contract it in the future (regarding the Gambler's Fallacy, see Pinkerton and Abramson 1992). They may continue to expose themselves—and perhaps others—to the danger of HIV infection and AIDS.

Promoting Testing to Women at Risk

Wishful Thinking

At present, wishful thinking lets people presume that they have been tested for HIV. Participants' discourse revealed that many view testing as part of a routine screening procedure (sometimes this is part of a dignity-preserving agreement between patient and omniscient practitioner). When a woman convinces herself that she need not specifically request an HIV test to get one, she can escape the embarrassment of having to verbalize her AIDS concerns to a clinician. Further, she can avoid having to think about the risks that she takes in her relationship(s); automatic testing implies nothing negative or frightening about a woman's lifestyle. All this, however, gets her no nearer to actually having been tested.

The Rule or the Exception?

As noted, women's status and self-esteem often depend on their relations with men and gain support from women's denial of AIDS risk and their related claims regarding honest fidelity. A woman must believe in her own wisdom and skill at choosing safe partners. She must trust her man when he says that he is true (and she must deny the significance of her own infidelities). To further support her beliefs or to bolster her social image when questioned, she may deny any need for testing.

Indeed, on the surface, HIV testing appears to obviate the Monogamy (and Wisdom) Narratives so many women tell. However, while a commitment to condom use expresses a relationship's fragility during every single protected sexual episode, having an HIV test is a special, infrequent occurrence. As such, it does much less to challenge monogamy beliefs than daily or otherwise regular condom use does. And as such, it can be cast as a method for checking up on a partner's escapades. It can be described as the smart choice made by the wise woman—the woman who acknowledges during a circumscribed moment that "you never really know" about your man's loyalty.

Better yet, an HIV test can be justified as a standard medical procedure. Indeed, talk about a partner's possible infidelities was often preceded by statements concerning the benefits of regular medical tests.

As Table 6 showed, five of the nine interviewees who had been tested and all four who had not yet gotten tested but desired to do so said that the test was (or would be) part of a routine examination. Twenty-six (70.3%) of the thirty-seven questionnaire respondents who claimed to have been tested and ten (62.5%) of the sixteen who wanted to get tested but who had not yet done so felt the same way.

Interviewees who anticipated having HIV tests were more likely to talk of the test's routine nature than those who had been tested previously, but this was not so for the questionnaire respondents. Interviewees may have invoked more talk of routine procedures because they felt more need than questionnaire respondents to present current relationships as intact and healthy: interviewees had to speak woman to woman with an interviewer and so had to worry about managing their self-presentations to a degree that questionnaire respondents did not. One's status and sense of self are more vulnerable in a face-to-face exchange, so strategic denial is even more important in the context of an interview or a clinic appointment. All of this suggests that screening policies that respect women's dignity, and their tendency to shift the testing discourse to one about normality when testing is decided on, will meet with more success than do current (humiliating) policies that equate testing with sociocultural deviance.

The AIDS and HIV Working Party of the Institute of Medical Ethics (IME) in the UK, mentioned above (Boyd 1990), came to the same conclusion, albeit by different means. The Party recommends "a policy of routine, but voluntary, diagnostic HIV testing" in which the HIV test is "offered as one of the normal antenatal tests" (177). The IME group favors "testing on an opting-out rather than an opting-in basis," so that "it is not left to the woman to make a positive request for it" (177).

An "opting-out" policy "may make it more difficult for a woman to say that she is not willing to have the test" (Boyd 1990, 177). However, the IME Party found this risk slight in comparison with the risk that "an opting-in policy might discriminate against those who were less articulate, or lacked background knowledge of HIV infection and its associated risks" (177). The implementation of an "opting-out" policy would both depend on and lead to the establishment of an environment in which HIV testing is neither stigmatized nor an indicator of stigma. And numerous inner-city U.S. women have already created a context-specific HIV test-related discourse describing such a world.

Because denying the possibility of unfaithfulness is so important for maintaining self-esteem and social status, trying to convince women to have HIV tests (or to use condoms) because their partners might not be monogamous is counterproductive. Clinicians know that beliefs about monogamy and gender roles make telling a woman that she should get an HIV test because she is promiscuous quite insulting. But they often fail to see that women—especially those who are socially and emotionally dependent on men—will be doubly insulted by the suggestion that their partners may be having extraconjugal sex. According to relationship ideals, men who do this do not really care about women's health and well-being.

The pain of admitting that your partner might not love or respect you is difficult to face. Rather than reminding women of their vulnerable position, clinicians might take a cue from their clients' own narratives about getting tested for HIV. Significantly, almost all the talk about infidelity was preceded or contextualized by talk about the routine nature of having any medical test at all, HIV tests included. Clinicians need to acknowledge this explanatory model, and to incorporate it into their HIV testing (and safer-sex) messages. The clinician-client relationship and the clinician's approach to testing have been shown to affect test uptake decisions (Bor et al. 1991; Meadows et al. 1990), so clinicians' adoption of approaches that appeal to normative cultural values and that enhance clients' self-esteem rather than damage it are essential.

Needless to say, a number of women and men do get tested. For many, test results are negative. Misinterpretations of the meaning of such results and their implications for sexual action, such as I described earlier in this chapter, must be guarded against by testing and counseling staff if testing is to be at all helpful for transmission prevention (cf. Kinsey 1994).

Other clients will test positive for HIV antibodies. Steps must be taken to improve the health care options available to impoverished HIV-positive people. Beyond guarding his or her health, the seropositive individual is faced with many other challenges, as Chapter 4 showed. One of the adjustments that the HIV positive are encouraged to make involves safer sex practice, both for primary prevention (in order to prevent the virus from spreading) and for secondary prevention (self-protection). This generally involves consistent condom use which, as we have seen, is not a simple matter. Sometimes, for the seropositive, condom use involves the added step of serostatus self-disclosure, and this makes safer sex all the more complex. The next chapter explores the issues that seropositive people face when dealing with self-disclosure to sexual partners.

    *   *   *

Much of the material in this chapter was adapted from "Attitudes Toward HIV Testing Among Inner-City Women," *Medical Anthropology* 16(2) (1994): 1–22.

Notes

1. While reading Ward's (1993b) paper, I found myself labeling the discourse of HIV-positive women "Betrayal Narratives." I noted how easily any of my own study's participants' stories might turn into a Betrayal Narrative if an HIV test came back positive. This influenced my conceptualization of the Monogamy Narrative and the Wisdom Narrative.

2. As Anderson and colleagues (1992) report in regard to 1989 NHIS data, the category of people "at increased risk" includes anyone who reported (1) being born in Haiti or in Central or East Africa, and anyone who reported that since 1977 she or he had (2) received blood products for hemophilia, (3) taken part in illicit injecting drug use, (4) participated in male homosexual activity, (5) participated in sex with anyone in groups one through four, or (6) sold or traded sex.

3. See Chapter 2, note 11.

4. As data were missing for one woman in this group, N = 52.

5. As mentioned, HIV test data were not collected from second-phase interviewees so that financial and social network data could be focused on.

6. Three of the nine interviewees who had been tested did cite their own high-risk practices when discussing their reasons for having gotten tested. But two of these three spoke of personal risk-taking in the context of talk of past drug use (i.e., habits not currently engaged in) and their partners' unsafe habits. The remaining woman was the only one in the group of nine pointing to her own sexual behavior as her primary reason for testing.

7. As the 1989 NHIS relied on self-reports, some participants may have erroneously believed themselves to have been tested when they had not been. The remainder of this chapter explores the various dimensions of that element of error. Mistaken testing reports might have been much greater for the study participants, in that their self-reported testing rates are much higher than even the "at increased risk" NHIS rates presented later in this section. This might have been because the study data were collected between 1992 and 1993 rather than in 1989, when the NHIS data were collected. The social desirability of testing seems to have increased over that time. Furthermore, real rates of testing have probably gone up, and the data from this study would reflect that increase. Testing increases are discussed in the note below.

8. It is important to note that these testing figures include blood donors who donated with HIV testing in mind. It also is important to note that they are three to four years older than the data that this book concerns. Results from the 1992 data set have just become available (Schoenborn et al. 1994). If we exclude blood-donation testing, 29 percent of Blacks were tested in 1992; otherwise, the frequency is 36 percent. Excluding blood-donors, 16 percent of whites were tested; including them, the figure is 18 percent. The base testing frequency for all U.S. adults regardless of race was 18 percent. Including blood donors who donated blood with testing in mind, it becomes 21 percent, which is no different from the percent who reported having been tested at all in 1989. However, the 1989 to 1992 test-frequency increases for Blacks (18.3–36 percent), which may have to do with clinics' heightened interest in testing programs, are impressive. They should be kept in mind when reviewing the testing frequencies for those 1989 NHIS respondents deemed "at increased risk." Similar frequencies for the 1992 "at increased risk" group are not yet available but, in light of the noted increase, they will no doubt be higher than the 1989 figures provided.

9. See note 2.

10. That the figures for Blacks are in the 70s rather than 60s may reflect the respective data collection dates rather than ethnic differences. Data for Blacks are two years older than the general data presented.

11. The frequency of testing for Blacks was actually slightly lower in "high-risk" cities than nationally: nationally, 30 percent of Black men and 24 percent of Black women had gotten tested; in "high-risk" cities, 27 percent of Black men and 23 percent of Black women had gotten tested. Regarding recent increases in testing among Blacks, see notes 8 and 10.

12. According to results from the National Health Interview Survey (Anderson et al. 1992), about one in five U.S. citizens has taken a voluntary HIV-antibody test and about one in ten, or half of those tested, have recollections of receiving post-test counseling. However, it is not clear how many of those who did not report receiving post-test counseling (if any) also did not receive the results of their tests.

13. An adjusted test-uptake frequency can be derived by multiplying the number of women who reported being tested but who did not recall being counseled (N = 10) by 43 percent (my estimate of the frequency with which counseling does *not* occur in tandem with testing in the United States, which is itself based on my estimate of the frequency with which counseling does occur: 57 percent; see Henry et al. 1991; Freeman 1991). The product of this multiplication operation (4.3), which represents the number of women who might actually have been tested even without being counseled, is then added to the number of women who did recall being counseled (3) for a total of 7.3. The adjusted test-uptake frequency is thus 38.5 percent (N = 19). Another way to derive an adjusted test-uptake frequency would be to consider the three women who did remember having been counseled as the 57 percent (the estimate of the frequency with which counseling does occur) and to figure out just what number three is 57 percent of. That number turns out to be 5.26. If the latter represents the number of women actually tested, the test-uptake frequency would be 27.7 percent. I have elected to use the larger estimated test-uptake frequency (38.5 percent) because I would rather give more women the benefit of the doubt. In any case, both estimates are purely speculative.

14. Similar beliefs and claims were reported by the inner-city youths participating in a study of sexual decision-making and attitudes toward AIDS among adolescents that I conducted with Dr. Gregory Zimet and Case Western Reserve Medical School's University Center for Adolescent Health's Sexuality Subcommittee (Zimet et al. 1995).

Chapter 9
Self-Disclosure Self-Described

The need for safer sex practice does not end with a negative HIV test; neither does it end with a positive diagnosis. Indeed, safer sex is as imperative for HIV-positive individuals as it is for HIV-negative individuals, not only because the former might otherwise pass the virus on but also because they are at risk for reinfection and for infection with other kinds of pathogens. While this project did not originally concern the experiences of individuals who know themselves to be HIV-positive, it soon became clear that, in addition to self-esteem and status-related concerns, the risk-related behavior of seronegative and untested people can be affected by the imagined threat of being lied to or manipulated by treacherous seropositive individuals.

Data from the few existing studies of self-disclosure (reviewed in Chapter 4) suggest that non-disclosure is indeed a problem. It may in many cases be motivated by desires for intimacy and fears of rejection. This chapter explores these desires and fears. Further, this chapter shows that for seropositive people non-disclosure also can be a rational strategy and a response to AIDS-risk denial in seronegative partners and those who do not know their serostatus. The apparent ubiquity of safer-sex information enables such non-disclosure by creating a sociocultural world in which risk taking by seronegative (or untested) individuals can be understood by seropositive people as stemming from well-informed decisions. Moreover, as standard safer-sex education messages suggest that when precautionary measures are taken all will be well, seropositive individuals may choose to keep their seropositivity secret while endeavoring to render the act of omission or non-disclosure harmless through prophylactic measures.

Background

Existing Knowledge

As noted in Chapter 4, self-disclosure among women has received little, if any, direct attention. It is mentioned in passing by Anitra Pivnick (1993) in a paper concerning the meaning of condoms among women attending a methadone clinic, twenty-two of whom were HIV positive (17.5%, N = 126). Sixteen of the twenty-two were married; fourteen of these women (87.5%) told their partners about their positive test results; two kept that information secret. But both of the women who had not self-disclosed insisted that their partners use condoms with them. Rather than say that this was because of HIV, they both told their partners that the condoms were for contraception.[1]

The protective action taken by the two non-disclosing married women suggests that portions of the standard safer-sex message are being drawn on by some people in a way that actually justifies non-disclosure. Both non-disclosing women doggedly followed standard safer-sex advice ("use a condom"), apparently with the assumption that this was sufficient means to protect their partners. Both this assumption and other possible factors contributing to non-disclosure must be examined, and we must ask whether women in other regions, or in other social groups, or who are not married[2] ever act similarly. Moreover, do men? The answer to the latter question holds great importance for women involved in heterosexual relations. A full inquiry is called for.

In order to gain insight into the little studied seropositivity self-disclosure process, and to illuminate the statistics generated by the epidemiological and quantitative projects reviewed in Chapter 4, I initiated a qualitative pilot study of the topic. The study also examined the possibility that the kind of AIDS-risk denial that I have described—or processes akin to it—intrude on the process of seropositivity self-disclosure. The research, which is exploratory, used focus groups in which the issues surrounding self-disclosure were submitted for discussion by HIV-positive people. Some interviews also were arranged to accommodate those who desired them.

Participants were drawn from the Southwest rather than the Midwest[3]; nonetheless, the HIV-positive individuals whose experiences I shall describe are similarly disadvantaged by poverty. I do not claim that their attitudes and intentions are representative, or that these can be generalized to the Cleveland group. However, as with the AIDS-risk denial examined in preceding chapters, I do suggest that the attitudes and intentions to be described are not especially unique. Indeed, some of the practices I shall describe are quite reminiscent of those reported for the non-disclosers in Pivnick's urban research (1993). While the attitudes and intentions of the Southwesterners are no doubt influenced to some degree by local conditions and by each person's life history, I suspect that future research will confirm my suggestion that their attitudes and intentions have much in common with those held by other HIV-positive people in the USA.[4]

Study Setting and Methods

The study was based at two southern New Mexico agencies offering services to HIV-infected people and PWAs.[5] Recruitment was carried out by mail. Each of agency one's forty-three and agency two's twenty-five local area clients was sent a small packet containing a brief demographic survey, a stamped envelope with my university address, and a letter explaining the plan — and the need — for the study.[6]

The response rate for agency one was 35 percent (n = 15). This is favorable when compared with the 21 percent response rate for another researcher's counseling survey sent out to the same group, and when compared to general response rates of between 20 and 25 percent for the regional agency's survey mailings (T. Call, personal communication). The response rate for agency two, for which no comparison statistics were available, was 40 percent (n = 10).[7]

Of the twenty-five individuals in total who responded, about half (n = 12) were able to participate.[8] Of the twelve, ages ranged from late twenties to mid forties.[9] The average monthly income (after taxes) was $562.75. Half the participants (n = 6) had AIDS.

As Table 7 shows, the sample consisted of five women and seven men. Although my focus has been on women's experiences, it is important to attend to what the men have to say. This is true even though most of the men who participated were not heterosexual. Many women have sex with bisexual (and sometimes wholly gay) men, whether or not these women know it.

Three men and five women participated in the focus groups. Three of the women and two of the men volunteered that they were ex-IDUs. (Because the pool of potential participants was so limited,[10] no effort was made to hold separate focus groups based on factors such as drug use history, age, infection duration, mode of transmission, sexual orientation, ethnicity, or relationship status.) One of the men was married to one of the women participating. A second, who was bisexual, also was married but he was experiencing difficulties with his wife and did not practice monogamy. No similar information was available for the third male participant, but his comments suggested that he was gay and single. Of the women, three were involved in steady heterosexual relationships. A fourth was in a steady homosexual relationship. However, she continued to engage in sex with men. The fifth woman was married but separated and so considered herself single. Her estranged husband was bisexual, as was a past long term partner of one of the other women.

To allow individuals who could or would not attend the focus groups but who wanted to help with the research a chance to participate, and to collect further information from three focus group participants who

TABLE 7. Participant Profiles

	Focus groups (N=8)	Interview only (N=4)	Total sample (N=12)
Sex			
Male	3	4	7
Female	5	0	5
Ethnicity			
Hispanic	2	3	5
Black	2	0	2
White	4	0	4
Asian	0	1	1
Conjugality			
Partnered	6	0	6
Single	2	4	6

were eager to provide it, seven private interviews were arranged.[11] The concerns of the interview-only participants (n = 4) were found to be similar to those of both the focus-group only (n = 5) and the focus-group-and-interview (n = 3) participants.

As Table 7 shows, all four of the interview-only participants were male. None of the interview-only participants was partnered; only one was sexually active. Two said that they preferred gay sex; one said that he was bisexual; one said that he was "normal" (heterosexual) but qualified this by adding that people frequently took him as gay because of his exaggeratedly "feminine" ways. So, whether in appearance or actuality, none of the interview-only participants was heterosexual. However, at least five of the eight focus-group participants were.

The focus groups met at agency offices in the early evenings, after hours. Copies of the mailed information letter and demographic survey were provided. Informed consent was verbally given. Discussions were audiotaped, with permission, and participants were paid for their time. The same procedures were followed with interviewees, who were interviewed at their convenience, in locations of their own choosing (generally, their homes).

Presentation of Findings

As mentioned in Chapter 5, one of the reasons for holding focus groups when in-depth ethnographic research is impossible is to allow the ethnographer access to detailed narrative data on intersubjectively held understandings regarding a given topic (cf. Schwartz 1978). Such data bespeak key dimensions of the intracultural debate surrounding the topic under question and provide information on the dialogical contexts in which specific kinds of responses will be provoked.

Certain dimensions of the debates surrounding seropositivity self-disclosure already have been discussed in Chapter 4, and so for the most part the participants speak for themselves in the sections that follow. When appropriate, focus group discourse is presented as conversation in order to preserve vital contextual information and to convey the key dimensions of the intersubjective debates carried on; other times, single speakers are quoted (pseudonyms are used in all cases[12]). Participants' own first-hand reports contain a depth of feeling and knowledge that my authorial voice can only partially and distortedly convey.

Discussions and interviews wove back and forth around five basic topics: (a) a disclosee's need to know about one's seropositivity, (b) the moral status of non-disclosure without and with safer sex practice (c) disbelief and denial among the seronegative, (d) strategies for evaluating potential disclosees, and (e) normalcy and acceptance versus rejection. Much conversation contained threads of a number of these topics. Notwithstanding, segments presented are grouped according to the five major themes.

A Disclosee's Need to Know

Most participants at first expressed the opinion that self-disclosure was necessary with sexual partners, and then qualified their statements by noting that this only was so if the partners in question were long term. For example, Maria said, "It's just — if you don't tell him and he gets the virus then you're really in deep shit." She explained:

If your partner doesn't know. . . . [Say] I'm with a man, and we've been in a relationship for years, I'm not cheating on him, he's not — we're not going out on each other: we're together. I have my tubes tied. It's not like I can get pregnant, so if I don't tell this guy he's not going to want to use a condom, and in the process he can get the virus from me, so of course by me telling him, he doesn't brush his teeth before we have sex — I mean there's a lot of little precautions that [we] take, including using a condom. On the norm [without a seropositive partner], you brush your teeth, you gargle, slap on a little cologne, "Let's go to bed." That's basically how it works. . . . But there are cautions that [we have to] take.

Participants agreed that long term partners have a need to know about one's seropositivity, especially because of the assumptions expressed by Maria that (a) monogamy renders AIDS risks null and void when neither partner is known to be seropositive, and (b) among heterosexuals, condoms can only be legitimately used in a monogamous relationship for contraception (Monogamy Narratives were discussed in Chapter 7). Participants also agreed that the last thing that they wanted was to infect others. Jon self-disclosed to his ex-partner "the day I found out because it's just—it's just my responsibility. I wouldn't put anybody's life in jeopardy for my own good." Max said, "By saying nothing, you risk their lives." Earlier, Max had said that non-disclosure was "not fair to the other person. Why put the other person through what [you] are going through?"

Three participants felt certain that HIV was "given" them by particular individuals: one of these participants was raped; the other two were married to non-disclosing bisexual men.[13] All three felt great fury in relation to their infections, which they had no control over stopping. One participant put it simply: "I had rage."[14] After being diagnosed, Janie self-disclosed to her estranged husband but only " 'cause I was angered. Because . . . he has never told me [about his bisexuality]. . . . It was more of an 'I want to get back at you' thing."

Dee described her partner's reaction to her own self-disclosure: "He's telling me to drop dead and how he was going to kill me." While such might keep many from self-disclosing, Dee felt that "It was urgent to get the news out . . . I wanted to stop him before he moved on [and spread the HIV] because I felt like this is my train—I started this train moving . . . I felt like I deserved whatever he would do to me 'cause I know the kill was the overkill." But no trains were derailed: after her partner "got over that level [i.e. of violent fury]," the two "went back in our tracks and asked people, 'Go get a test; it's free at Planned Parenthood.' [And they say,] 'I don't want to know.' " Janie's estranged husband acted similarly: "Up to this day he knows about it but he will not get checked . . . He says he don't have it, period." The benefits of disclosing when the response is such seem minimal, especially in comparison with the high costs of rejection and the very real threat of physical attack.

The Moral Status of Non-Disclosure
Without and With Protection

Several participants thought that many seropositive people use non-disclosure coupled with unsafe sex to express their rage. "People are going out and doing this stuff on purpose," Dee explained. "They [say,] 'Well somebody gave it to me so I'm going to give it to someone else.' That's horrible. That's murder to me."

Ron told of a seronegative friend who said to him,

"If I found out I had that, I'd be out there trying to get [i.e., infect] every [woman] I could." He looked at me with a straight face and told me this, like I'd be so angry so mad at the world that I'd just go out and try and—I believe there are more people out there doing that than you would really believe . . . [They] just point blank don't even think about it anymore except for the fact that they want to take somebody with them.

In telling such stories — in contrasting themselves with such "horrible" people — Dee and Ron and the others present themselves as morally upright and highly ethical. This may be a method of self-esteem preservation. As Ron explained, "Low self-esteem is a constant thing with many people who've had this disease," which "is the biggest shit that we could be in." Prior to his own diagnosis, he said, he was plagued by the idea that he had not fulfilled his family's expectations; "I [thought I was] this wretched human being." The need to defend one's reputation by telling tales of even more "wretched" individuals is manifest.

Amidst the moralizing rhetoric, Rick confessed to having had unsafe sex without self-disclosing, just like the hyperbolized serial HIV killer does. But, he noted,

I don't think I was necessarily having unsafe sex to hurt anybody. . . . When you're doing drugs you do all kind of — your reasoning is pretty much gone. . . . I reasoned it that the person that I was with probably already was infected, and I was in fact right, but it didn't . . . that doesn't make it right.

Rick's move from presenting himself as a man lacking reason to one having fine logic capabilities bothered no one as the two claims, so differently contextualized, made sense independently.

Joe, who is married, also told of non-disclosure. But for Joe, who is bisexual and who kept his condition from his wife (as well as from others, more of which later), time was the issue. He said that he meant to inform her but had not yet done so when she found out.[15] Fear of exposing their homosexuality or bisexuality (and sometimes their unfaithfulness) to female lovers causes many closeted men to hide their seropositivity (e.g., Chiodo and Tolle 1992, Dunbar and Rehm 1992, Gard 1990). If Joe had such a fear, he did not mention it. But the possibility of raising accusations of such was a big issue for Max, who held that when people learn that a man is seropositive, they immediately ask themselves, Eric summarized: " 'Is he gay? . . . Does he sleep around? Is he a big whoredog? Does he do drugs?' Disclosing to somebody is like sewing a scarlet letter on."

Maria kept her serostatus secret from a number of partners, but this was conjoined with safe sex practice. She explained, "I was in and out of monogamous relationships and I'd never told them, you know? I protected, 'cause I didn't want to catch anything else, but I also knew that if I was with a man that I would protect him." In addition to sending a message regarding beneficent or altruistic safer sex practice in this statement ("I protect him"), Maria used the designation "monogamous" to confer sociocultural legitimacy on short term relationships, and she voiced her concern for her own health in addition to that of her partners. Regarding the latter, she noted:

What people don't realize is that *we* catch things. And they're so scared of catching stuff from us. You know, a common cold can kill me? I mean, people don't realize that. And some people just totally freak, and [loud whisper] "Oh my god she's HIV positive!" and "She has AIDS!" And they're coughing all over me and gossiping at the same time. And I'm thinking, "Don't you know that cold can kill me?"[16]

One's physical self-protection notwithstanding, a relationship's duration and character seem to be key to self-disclosure decisions. As Dee, who insisted on telling her partner, pointed out, "Who's going to tell a one-night stand anyway? Nobody's going to tell them." This is because it is not deemed necessary for the good of the relationship, and because the consequences of telling a new or one-time partner, who does not necessarily have one's best interests in mind, could be dire. Almost all participants promoted non-disclosure conjoined with sexual safety measures in such situations.

Participants felt that the strategy of beneficent prophylaxis (i.e., the benevolent insistence on safer sex) would negate a partner's need to know about one's seropositivity.[17] As Joe said, "I would not disclose, but I would make sure there were no dangers [by taking] safety measures." Maria related a story:

"We're driving home from the bar [after I met] this guy . . . And I says to [my friend, the driver], "Should I tell him I'm HIV positive? I'm gonna sleep with this guy." And he's like, "I don't think you should." I says, "Well, maybe I should." He says, "Just use a condom. Just make sure you use a condom. You're not going to get in a relationship with this guy—he's married." And I thought, "OK." So I slept with him, I have been sleeping with him. . . . But we always looked—every time I go to [Meg's] house, [I ask her to] give me a couple of condoms, just in case. I have condoms in my pocket when I go out to the bars, see, and I never told him. And it's about a month and half later and, yeah, I guess I'm cheating on my old man [laughter]. But I protected [the bar guy]."

Interestingly, the friend who suggested non-disclosure coupled with safer sex was seronegative. Similarly, Dee said, "[People] tell me, 'Girl, if I was you I wouldn't tell!' "

Maria remarked that she sometimes felt guilty for withholding serostatus information but, she said, in relation to the tale above, "You know what? The guy turned out to be a real asshole anyway." A health care worker who had been fired and who knew the man Maria was dating "told this guy that I was HIV positive. And the guy confronted me with it, and I denied it. I totally denied it, and he said, 'Well, if you had AIDS, you know, I would kill you.' . . . But I never put him at risk."

The prospect of bodily harm may make many women hesitant to self-disclose to male partners. But for now, my focus is on Maria's point regarding prophylaxis. Similar statements came from most participants describing sex with casual partners. Janie proclaimed, "I don't say, but I do take precautions," Rick declared. "I don't tell, but [I do] protect." People were not always so punctilious in actuality:

Maria: You can't sleep with someone [without protection] and then say, "Hey, by the way, I'm HIV positive." It just doesn't work that way—
Joe: It does too.
Maria: Well, it doesn't work for me.
Joe: I've done it, I mean I've slept with a person —
Maria: And then tell him you're HIV?
Joe: Mmm-hmm [yeah].
Maria: How did they react?
Joe: Same. Actually I was very very much surprised by the reaction. . . . I started to feel guilty that I'm not telling the other person that I'm HIV positive and so I told the other person that I was, and that didn't change the circumstances [i.e., they didn't use condoms, etc.]

Disbelief and Denial Among the Seronegative

Many participants said that despite high levels of AIDS awareness among the lay public (and high knowledge levels exist even among the disenfranchised; see, e.g., Harrison 1991; Jemmott and Jemmott 1991) partners often choose to forgo protection. Participants sometimes understood this as stemming from uncounterable stupidity. Ron argued, "Human beings are human beings and they're still going to do the same stupid shit that got us into this shit anyway." Earlier, he said, "We don't learn from history," and noted, "We're like any other animal but probably with a few more problems, because of the so-called free will that we think we have."

While Ron did not believe in free will, many of the other participants felt that as AIDS knowledge is high (or perceived to be so) a partner's refusal to use condoms must stem from informed personal choice:

Maria: The majority of people know about AIDS. The majority of people know about how they can get it. If you're going to pick somebody up in a bar, that guy might have it, or that girl might have it. I'm gonna protect myself from that person. . . .
Joe: But haven't you run into a situation where they may know but they may not care?
Maria: Yeah, I have.

Joe: I mean, there's that point. I mean, people are educated to some degree about HIV and AIDS. It is how that person reacts and how that person acts to protect him- or herself with the other partner, and although they may know, they'll take the risk anyway.

Maria: That's true, that's very true.

Joe: So I mean if at that point in time—It just depends, I have said that sometimes I do [tell] and sometimes I don't. When I have [told and] the other person knows full well and they choose not take any safety measures, that decision is totally up to them. That's their decision.

Likewise, Janie said, "If a person's willing to have sex and just do it . . . OK" [i.e., that's their decision]. But Eric said that you "can't assume somebody else's knowledge [and so you have] to accept responsibility [i.e., insist on protection]."[18]

Some participants explained condom refusal as based in denial, a term that they use as if self-explanatory[19]:

Rick: I've had people say to me, "Well, you don't have AIDS; you don't need to use a condom." I said "Regardless of what I am, you would use a condom wouldn't you?"

Dee: In this day and age!

Janie: [concurrently] You would think so.

Rick: [They say,] "Well what's wrong?" I mean I've been through it. . . . I thought to myself, "I don't know if I want to have sex with this person after all." Not only are they loose, but . . . [I had decided that] I'm going to really make an effort to use this—do the safe stuff . . . Sometimes it's the other side! You'll negotiate and then it's like—it gets to be sort of a hassle.

Dee: The think we too healthy to have AIDS. If you're overweight you don't have anything.

Ron: You've got to be skinny, have your hair falling out or something.

Dee: I tell them, "You don't realize! You need to get more educated on that subject . . . " I have said to people, "Why do you want to be with me? For all you know I got AIDS!" [And they say,] "Oh look at you: all them big thighs! You don't have any AIDS." They're in denial.

Max's strategy for countering condom refusal was similar to Dee's and Rick's, with mention of condoms' contraceptive benefits thrown in.

As Ron said, despite one's protestations, "It's very difficult to negotiate for safe sex." Janie agreed: "It's not easy, because my partner—well, my partner doesn't like using condoms, and I get afraid because I know the importance of it, and yet he doesn't, so he doesn't seem to see." (Many participants did not like using condoms themselves. As Ron explained, "They're really so nasty.") Later, Janie explained,

They don't like using condoms, and right off the bat they say, "Well I don't have AIDS." That's the first thing: "I don't have AIDS." And I go, "I didn't say you did," and then they say, "I had myself checked two months ago" [which shows that they really do not understand the disease] but you don't want to go into detail with them, because by that time they wonder, "Well why are you so up to date on that stuff?"

Maria pointed out, "Most men do not accept women being HIV-positive. It's a difficult thing for them, I guess because it's [perceived as] a gay disease."

According to participants, besides failing to internalize the safer sex message and so denying their own risks for AIDS (see Chapters 3, 7, and 8), people also harbor disbelief when disclosed to. In a statement that bears out findings regarding pregnancy among HIV-positive women (reviewed in Chapter 2; see also Arras 1990; Levine and Dubler 1990; Pivnick et al. 1991), Maria said,

I found out [I was HIV positive], and I got pregnant. I was perfectly healthy. I took that chance and had that baby and he was perfectly healthy. . . . And [my ex-partner], through the whole entire time, did not believe me; for years, never believed me. "Ah, you're full of it." He'd always tell me that. He didn't believe me and we never protected each other and I kept always telling him and then I ended up getting pregnant, and he didn't believe me until the guy who takes the blood—what are they called? He came in to draw my blood and he put two pairs of gloves on and [my ex] says, "Why you wearing all those gloves" " 'Cause she's HIV positive." [My partner's] eyes got this big around! I mean, he was sitting in his chair and he was like [sits straight up] "What?!" And just jumped out of his chair, and I looked at him, and I said, "What? Do you think I've been lying to you for six years? I've been telling you for years."

Strategies for Evaluating Potential Disclosees

Deciding whether, when, and how to self-disclose is seen as based on a special kind of intuition. Joe explained, "You start to develop a judgment call type of thing . . . Your senses become more sharpened." He and the others described a pattern like one that Barbara Limandri (1989) described for self-disclosing stigmatizing conditions in general: the disclosee's responses to small bits of information are evaluated as the discloser searches for a sign that a full revelation will not result in rejection. Max explained, "You can't just explode it to everybody or they'll run away."

Dee said, "You go at them one way and you see, 'Well, that's not going to work. I can't do that. I got to regroup and come back with this.' " Gloria advised, "You feel it out, you know. You wait and see, 'cause in conversation you can hear what people are open to and what they're closed off to . . . You can spot narrow minds and closed minds; you can, just it shows."

The duration and depth of the relationship in question seems key.

Janie said that in the case of a one-night stand, "You don't know the person, [you don't know if] when they go home, are they gonna say [anything]? What are they gonna say? Where they gonna say it? To who? You don't want that [i.e., gossip]." A casual partner's potential role as a gossip was horrifying to Janie, whose whole family had learned of her illness through the grapevine. Still, as she knew, people often cannot help talking; when Janie told one confidante, "it affected her and she had to tell [someone else] so she could help herself."

Others also warned that one should not self-disclose until a relationship had solidified. Eddie said that the time to self-disclose was when partners decided to make commitments to each other as lovers. Joe said, "I would not disclose at first to anybody . . . until that relationship had time to build so that you had something to disclose to."

Participants did not seek self-disclosure advice from counselors but from other seropositive individuals if at all. In part, this was due to negative counseling experiences at the time of initial diagnoses. As Maria said, "I went down to the health department, and they just kinda, 'OK, here, by the way you're HIV positive,' poofed me out the door." Meg got her diagnosis at a doctor's office, and she too received little in the way of guidance or support: "My doctor [just] gave me a bottle of — a prescription of Valium and told me to go home and take a couple and mellow out."

Overall, participants felt that local client services were lacking. "I almost get the feeling that they don't care," said Jon, adding:

I get the feeling that the people who are in charge are doing it just for a job . . . Everybody who works at [an agency in Northern New Mexico] is either gay or is positive in AIDS and they really care and they really help you out . . . Here, one time I went in and I was waiting in the lobby to see somebody and I was going through their magazine thing and I saw they had a local gay magazine and I went to pick it up and it was about six months old!

Max said of area counselors, "They're not talkable, you know? Or there's a lecture behind it." Positive comments did come from two of the heterosexual women without histories of drug use (suggesting the possibility of a bias on counselors' parts) but, overall, participants did not utilize area counseling services.[20]

Maria: I've never gone to see a counselor and said, "Listen, I'm in this relationship and I want to know if I should tell my lover or not, that I'm HIV."
Joe: I've gone to support groups, an HIV-positive support group.
Maria: That's how you find out what to do.
Meg: I shy away from support groups . . . I don't want to tell strangers that I've got HIV.
Maria: But they're not strangers. We're all blood related — we're family.
Meg: Well I don't know these people, OK? And these people don't know me. . . .
Maria: I started going to the support groups when I very first came [home],[21] and

it was OK. And then it ended up with just me and some other guy and a gal who was supposed to open [the center] for us wouldn't show up and so it kinda just fell apart.

Janie had a similar story regarding support groups: she went to one only to find that "there's two people there in this group thing!" Although Janie blamed this on the agency's lack of "enthusiasm," low attendance might have been due to the fear of exposure that Meg alluded to above and that Janie summed up in remarks about the health-seeking process. She said, "When the volunteers help you, they look at you, and you go, 'Oh, God, now if you ever see me on the street you're going to know,' " and "You have to go get your prescription and then the pharmacist knows what this prescription is for, and . . . you go, 'Oh God, they know.' " And, as happened to Maria, sometimes they do tell.

Normalcy and Acceptance or Rejection

When asked whether most HIV-positive people self-disclosed to sexual partners, Max, who was not sexually active at the time of his participation, told me,

Most people pretend they don't have it . . . not on purpose, but to feel normal again. They want to stay with a healthy point of view rather than to be thinking about it all the time . . . Every day people are dying and so you try to stay with a positive attitude.

Max elaborated on the concept of retained or regained normalcy through non-disclosure by talking about HIV testing. With a positive result, he said, "you are so lost." Many people think that if they "take another blood test it won't be there; it was a mistake or misunderstanding."

Max said that HIV-positive people "go back to being normal" when "they pretend it's not there." Earlier, he spoke of a "human" desire for a "feeling of being not alone; feeling wanted." Non-disclosure appeared to Max as a way to gratify those desires, while in disclosing "you take the chance of them leaving. [But] you need the affection of somebody else other than family or friends. You are lonely, and scared you're gonna die." Similarly, Dee noted,

You found out you don't want to be by yourself. If you got somebody you're interested in or somebody is interested in you, you better hold on, because you're going to realize late at night, two or three o'clock in the morning — you get up and go to the bathroom and go back to bed and can't go to sleep — you're going to realize you just can't do it by yourself, you need [somebody].

Janie also talked about "wanting that attention in that manner and no one to have it [from]."

While Janie was actively seeking a steady relationship, six of the twelve participants were partnered at the time of the study. When describing her experience of disclosing to her primary partner, whom she met after being diagnosed, Maria said,

We dated for about two weeks and we were kinda getting close. It was really hard for me. "No, I'm not going to tell him yet; yeah I'll tell him; no I'm not going to tell him." And I thought, like, "I can't give it to him." And I went back and forth with it, and I just kinda started eating up inside about it. And then finally I just said "Hey, I'm HIV positive; how do you feel about this?" So he got out of the truck and went to the bathroom in the gas station and came back and he was just looking at me, like, "What?" "Well, I just told you something." "Oh, I love you, it's OK." I was like, "*What?*" I expected rejection. [Meg interjects: "So did I."] I really expected to be rejected, like, "Oh my God how can you do this?" Or, "Ooh I don't want to be a part of *that.*"

The fear of rejection is paramount, and the struggle to decide to disclose ("Yeah I'll tell him; no I'm not going to tell him") is clear.

"Acceptance and rejection. That's the two main issues," declared Maria. Rejection can come from within as well as from without: denial, shame, and anger are common responses at least in the initial weeks after diagnoses (Kurth and Hutchison 1989; McCain and Gramling 1992). Eric's hypothetical advice to partners of HIV-positive people, "Get out while you can," bespeaks such self-rejection.

The question of partnering with other seropositive people, who might be more sympathetic and with whom one might be able to be more candid, was raised in both focus groups by the participants. For example, Rick said, "I prefer—I feel better about it [partnering with seropositive individuals]. It's probably not better for you or anything [but] I feel more comfortable with it. I feel it gets that stuff out of the way. It is an issue still, but it's not like a big disclosure."

In the other group, the question was raised by Joe and taken up by Maria:

Joe: It think it is kinda chance [that I have not been with anyone who is HIV positive] because I was going, I was debating—
Maria: Would you be with someone?
Joe: Actually it may take some of the pressure off of me if I was involved with somebody who was actually HIV positive and we could deal with it in a healthier way instead of having to reserve [repress, keep secret] all my feelings, cause right now I do reserve all my feelings in relation to [my wife].

But partnering with a seropositive person did not seem smart to Maria, who explained:

I don't think I can have a relationship with someone that's positive, actually I couldn't. [It would be a] turn off. To me, I'm healthy; to me, I'm kinda normal. . . . And if I got into a relationship with someone else that was HIV positive my whole world would be HIV positive, because I got to deal with someone else that was HIV positive and I would have to deal with their issues about being HIV positive and I couldn't do that. . . . [Plus,] I would be scared of catching something! [laughter]

The question of partnering with seropositive people notwithstanding, the fear of rejection by the seronegative was paramount. Meg told her partner but, she said, "I was scared to, because I didn't know if he was going to leave me or if he was just gonna like stay with me for a little while and then leave or just leave me right then and there." He stayed. So did Jon's partner, who, Jon said, "was very supportive of me. We stayed together for quite a while."

Maria encountered rejection from neither her current primary partner nor from her past one:

You know, even after my [then-boyfriend] found out—I mean for sure *knew* that I was HIV positive, it still never mattered to him. This guy was so in love with me. His thing was, "If you're going to die, we'll die together." I thought, "That's the ultimate." Yeah. That's kinda like the Romeo and Juliet thing, you know. . . . [He stood by me], knowing still I was HIV positive. A lot of people go through the fact "I'm HIV positive I can never find another person."

Maria's statement bespeaks a fear that HIV seropositivity means an end to all intimacy if revealed, and it fits with the research conclusions described in the three preceding chapters regarding the significance of unsafe sex as symbolic of love and devotion. It also demonstrates that despite the fact that, as Maria said, "It can cost us for telling someone," there were stories of self-disclosure successes. As Meg said, in addition to herself, "There's people that I know who have told their partners and they're still in relationships."

Janie also mentioned role models, but although she felt encouraged by them, she had not disclosed to the man that she was dating. "I'm afraid that if he'd know he might not want to be with me or spend time with me," she said, explaining that she did not want to scare him away:

I don't have anybody to really be a mate, a companion; I don't have that. So when I think about it, it hurts. You just think that you don't have nothing to live for. . . . You say to yourself, "Are you ever going to be involved with anybody? Is anybody going to accept you? Are they going to want you once they find out? Are they going to have a life with you?"

Janie's words, like those reported earlier for Max, were a plea for normalcy.

Of the participants, only Dee and Joe reported rejection from a primary partner. In Joe's case, it was his wife, who learned of his condition from an outside source. Her rejection included temporarily cutting Joe off from his children, which Joe said left "a big crater in my heart that could not be filled no matter how you were to fill it."

Joe's wife's rejection lessened over time and patterns of interaction were reestablished as acceptance grew. The same was true for Dee. But in other cases, hurts did not mend. And, as Joe pointed out, rejection isn't always immediate: "When I chose to disclose to [a steady lover, he] would at first say it was OK, yet the more that [we were] in the relationship . . . there were other issues that came out, [from] down below." Joe's partner was slowly shutting down on him emotionally; he "was having a hard time . . . He felt 'I cannot love you because you are HIV positive; I cannot feel more than that.' And that's restricting."

Joe suggested that partners of seropositive people form a support group. "So, what if your partner doesn't want to go?" Meg asked. "That's their choice," Joe said, adding, "You cannot force that person." Partners who do not wish to participate are cast as their own masters, much as condom avoiders were in the earlier discussion of unsafe casual sex.

The interchange continued as Joe explained that self-disclosure often ignites a long process of emotional work in partners. His wife and he talk, Joe said, but only "surface talk, surface talk. They're going through their own set of issues. . . . They may have issues that they haven't totally [discovered] because it's a process, it's a learning process." Joe also said, "They will want to isolate you, they want you all to themselves. But they want to isolate you [also because] they don't want anybody else to know that you're HIV positive." Maria added, "They're embarrassed of the idea of a lover being HIV."

As Janie said, "You're trying to support yourself, but then you're going to have to support them." Concern for the disclosee can influence self-disclosure decisions.

Ron: When we disclose to somebody what we're afraid of [is that] we know what
        we went through having it, in a way they kinda go through it in their own
        little way too . . . They're like flipped out, and I think to myself, "You don't
        have this disease, I do.
Janie: They want sympathy.
Rick: No, but they do. You're more inclined to be more concerned for them
        [than for yourself].

Still, as Meg said, disclosure "takes emotional strain off of you. You got too much to worry about as it is."

Although not put forth as a topic for discussion, self-disclosure to children emerged as salient in both focus groups. Interview-only participants did not concern themselves with the issue, perhaps because neither they nor their past partners had children. But Janie's assertion, "Children are more supportive than I feel others would be. . . . Their minds are open to learn and understand," was typical of focus group members.

Of her own children, Janie said, "they see that I am a single parent, and I'm doing my best, and when they see that I'm tired or I'm this or that, they're there . . . and they take that extra time for me." When she was first diagnosed, Janie said, "I went into depression . . . [but] I kept working. I remembered that my kids — my mom kept saying, 'Your children will need you.' "

The importance of children's love is made clear in the following interchange, in which children are favorably compared to (fickle) adults.

Joe: When I [was estranged from my family and] didn't have my child around me for a long time, I said, "I want a baby." I wanted a baby so bad that — because a child will give you the love with no strings.

Maria: That's right. That's why I chose to have my son.

Joe: They don't give you — they will give you emphatic love without any question whatsoever.

Maria: Unconditional.

Joe: And for that rejection that I've felt — I needed, to recuperate for my own self-preservation, [I needed] a little bit of acceptance and a little bit of love that was *unconditional.* . . .

Maria: . . . Children love you without condition. They — children — my son: he's great. I really am grateful that I chose to have this child. You know, I was told that I had a thirty percent chance that this child would come out having the virus. I left it in God's hands and I tell you that this baby loves me. . . .

Joe: Children bring out — that's why I choose to live with my kids is because I get emotional support that for me can never be equaled in any way, shape, or form. And they'll be there for me until we all pass away. . . . Children . . . don't fish around, they don't pull any punches or at least —

Maria: They don't gossip about it: "Did you know," "What I really want to know is . . ."

Joe: . . . When you disclose to the children, and all of us have children in this room, it's — it's a healthy thing because nothing has changed in their perception of who you are. . . .

Meg: And children do help the partner to develop, 'cause they're so honest and they still love you. It helps that partner to see that. "The child loves her and I should too." Or, "Kids aren't scared, why should I be?"

Maria: . . . That child just loves you, just unconditionally, just to pour their hearts out to you always be there and always love you no matter how sick or how bad you look. That child will always love you, and that also gives a partner that other perspective. . . . Even my mother — my son has given my mom strength in learning to love me all over again . . .

Non-Disclosure and Murderous Intent?

Participants advocated self-disclosure on a need-to-know basis, and for most this hinged on the duration and depth of the relationship in question. Participants felt that beneficent prophylaxis removed the need to know in certain cases, such as with casual sex partners or when the threat of rejection meant that the cost of self-disclosing was likely to outweigh any benefit. The fact that many untested or seronegative individuals deny their own AIDS risks (for reasons discussed in the preceding chapters) sometimes made this a difficult strategy to implement.

The recommended method for evaluating the likelihood of being rejected by potential disclosees involved making indirect allusions to stigmatized lifestyles or conditions and then judging reactions. Participants noted that even those who accept their disclosures can harbor surreptitious fears or can make the acceptance conditional. Moreover, they can revoke or threaten to revoke it at later points in time, sometimes obliquely (as by using other issues as ruses for partial or complete rejection of the discloser).

As noted by participants, and as mentioned in Chapters 4 and 8, many people become angry on learning of their seropositivity. Fury and rage may turn a person rancorous and vindictive. When one does not know against what or whom to seek revenge — and in the case of AIDS it is frequently difficult to track down the route of transmission — any human target may do. But, generally, anger subsides and people move on to enter stage two of the coping process previously described (McCain and Gramling 1992), which involves fighting AIDS, not other people.

Rumors of vindictive people who prowl around town spreading HIV among unknowing innocents appeal to many because, one's serostatus notwithstanding, faced with the uncontrollable likes of the AIDS pandemic, urges run high to attribute blame, to scapegoat, to cast ourselves as victims, and to hunt out witches (cf. Farmer 1992).[22] Furthermore, a metaphoric connection between murderous, cunning non-disclosers and the murderous and seemingly cunning AIDS virus itself, which uses a kind of trickery to penetrate and insinuate itself into cells' reproductive systems, may be operating. In any case, and as noted in Chapter 3, people who feel defenseless against non-disclosers may fatalistically abandon caution in their sexual encounters.

People do keep their seropositivity a secret from sexual partners in many cases, as the studies reviewed and the data just presented show. However, the idea that many people do so in order to cause harm (i.e., in order to infect others) and the notion that some people actively use their HIV-positive bodies as lethal weapons (e.g., by spewing bodily fluids on those whom they would harm) probably have more to do with public paranoia and the media sensationalism that feeds this than they have to do with fact (see also Chapter 3).

Intervention Implications

In a letter to the editor of the *Journal of the American Medical Association,* Kegeles et al. write, in reference to their own research, that "A sizable minority of people engaging in sexual activities may transmit HIV [do] not intend to tell their partners," whether primary or secondary, about their serostatus (1988, 217). Kegeles et al. further note that these findings "underscore the need for sexually active individuals to protect their health by following 'safe sex' practices, since not all sexual partners can be depended on to be forthright about their antibody status" (217).

Despite the fact that not all HIV-positive individuals self-disclose, particularly to casual or secondary partners, study findings support other data indicating that many seropositive people do increase safer-sex practices (see also Cleary et al. 1991; Kelly et al. 1989; Wykoff et al. 1988). Further, findings support the conclusion that self-disclosure and safer sex are not the same thing; the former does not necessarily entail the latter (Perry et al. 1994, 1990). Safer sex must be promoted to HIV-positive individuals, their self-disclosure behaviors notwithstanding. Not only should sexual partners be protected, as with condoms, but the health of HIV-positive individuals themselves should be guarded through proactive efforts. The theme of self-protection that surfaced in participants' discourse could be exploited.

While safer sex is the best protection against infection, it is not foolproof: HIV could still be spread. HIV-positive individuals must be informed and reminded of this fact. Such knowledge can encourage self-disclosure because it can increase the need to know that the seropositive individual will attribute to potential sex partners. Information regarding the mechanisms of denial among the seronegative, as are described in this book, can also encourage self-disclosure in this fashion. That is, if counselors remind HIV-positive people that others often fail to internalize AIDS prevention knowledge, and that, for example, others often think that choosing only partners that they see as "safe" (as by appearance) is enough to protect against HIV transmission (even though apparently "safe" partners may be HIV-positive), then HIV-positive individuals may not be so quick to accept an initial reluctance to practice safer sex on a partner's part as an informed choice. The HIV-related altruism indicated by the reported frequency with which the individuals described here attempt beneficent prophylaxis, as well as by other research, especially with women (Kline and VanLandingham 1994) but also with men (Solomon and DeJong 1989), can be tapped into as HIV-positive people are provided counseling in regard to methods for persuading partners to take precautionary measures (skills training interventions are mentioned in Chapter 10; see also Taylor and Lourea 1992; Valdiserri et al. 1989; Vander Linden 1993).

Regarding the self-disclosure process, counselors can encourage clients to test potential disclosees with strategic invitational advances. John Green (1989) encourages counselors and clients to practice self-disclosing through role playing. It is important, notes Green, that clients sometimes play the role of the partner being disclosed to in order to gain an understanding of the feelings this entails. If the situation warrants it, counselors may point out that, as this research indicates, many people have self-disclosed with positive results. However, counselors should prepare clients for possible future traumas by noting that rejection can lurk below acceptance, as it did for Joe. Counselors might encourage self-disclosure to partnered clients who have children, as children can encourage disclosed-to partners to be more accepting (they can also provide support and a sense of purpose to self-disclosers).

Two recommendations regarding counseling also can be made based on these findings. First, clients seem to have trouble absorbing information provided in the post-test setting. McCann and Wadsworth (1991) studied the experience of testing in a clinic in which post-test counseling was the policy and found that two in five (41%, N = 252) seropositive people did not remember receiving AIDS information when they received their test results. This "raises questions about how much can be achieved immediately after a test result is given" (52), when testees' assimilation capacities may be minimal. Although discussion of partner notification issues (as well as of other issues) was supposed to have occurred in post-test counseling where this chapter's research took place, participants did not recall any such discussion. Partner notification must therefore be broached during later contact sessions as well. This means that great efforts must be taken to ensure future encounters with clients, who all to often, it seems, abandon counseling early on. The second recommendation follows from this.

For clients to use available counseling services more fully, they must be made to feel welcome. Staff members should make special efforts to carry out duties as if these are elected tasks that have expressive or moral value. HIV counseling cannot be viewed as just a job that leads to a pay check. Clients who sense staff members' lack of commitment or tendency to lecture will turn away.[23] Also, staff members must make efforts to compensate for possible oversensitivity on clients' parts.

The data here presented, which begin to make up for the dearth of qualitative information concerning seropositivity self-disclosure, have policy implications. So do the risk-denial data presented in the preceding chapters. More ideas about just how AIDS educators can encourage safer sex are discussed in the next, and final, chapter.

Notes

1. Also participating in Pivnick's study (1993) were seropositive unmarried women with lovers. No information regarding the reasoning or the specific safer sex practices of these women was provided, although it was suggested that they often used condoms.

2. See note 1.

3. The research site change came about because of my own relocation from Case Western Reserve University in Cleveland to New Mexico State University.

4. The research does have limitations, especially in light of the fact that the self-selection process recruitment entailed may have introduced certain biases into the data. Persons responding to the call to participate acknowledge their sero-positivity and feel comfortable or at least willing to discuss their private concerns with or in front of a stranger. Also, some of the participants in the focus groups knew each other already (considering how few seropositive individuals live in the region, this would be expected). This may have promoted self-protective secrecy; it also may have kept the involved participants from spinning tales and have led them to introduce certain topics for discussion that otherwise might have been skipped (at times, for example, one person would correct the other or ask a specific question of her or him; regarding focus group methods, see Bender and Ewbank 1994; VanLandingham et al. 1994). Further, Las Cruces, which is the biggest town in southern New Mexico, and which was the research site, is actually quite small (pop. 65,000). HIV-positive citizens understandably fear having relatives, neighbors, or co-workers see them enter local health agency offices. Despite the presence of a university, Las Cruces is not at all cosmopolitan. The town's seal depicts three Christian-style crosses and a citizens' prayer meeting was recently held in government offices. Faculty parking stickers were pink triangles at the time the research was done; most people in Las Cruces were blind to the significance of this symbol except insofar as it reveals a bit about the occupation of the stickered car's owner. The perceived threats entailed in participating in an HIV/AIDS-related project in such an atmosphere, despite the promise of confidentiality and anonymity, must be intense (a similar reluctance to participate in research held by individuals living in a similarly provincial region is reported in Laryea and Gien 1993).

5. Megan McGuire and David Simonsmeier were instrumental in facilitating the research. Dorothy Ball, Terry Call, Carl Valles, and Gail Wheeler also helped with the project at different times.

6. I prepared the mailings, which were given to an agency staff member who had access to the roster and so could make mailing labels without compromising the anonymity and confidentiality concerns of the clients. I explained this process to clients in the letter so that they would know their names and addresses were unknown to me.

7. Agency two had only just begun serving HIV-positive people.

8. Often, non-participation was explained as due to failing health.

9. There are so few HIV-positive individuals in the region that to provide real ages might compromise participants' anonymity. For the same reason, certain

biographical facts that might have illuminated the personal meanings of some of the discourse reported have been left out.

10. Southern New Mexico is a rural region with low population density. While New Mexico had reported a total of 861 AIDS cases by the end of 1993, only 81 of those came from southern counties, and only 32 from the Las Cruces region (NMHDU 1994: 10). The relative dearth of AIDS cases in southern New Mexico is matched by the relative paucity of HIV-positive people on official lists (according to regional HIV/AIDS workers, many HIV-positive individuals in this region, particularly if moneyed, avoid public services because of confidentiality concerns). See also note 21 and regarding methodological limitations, see note 4.

11. This is not to say that the other five focus group participants were uninterested in interviews; arrangements were problematic, as they often will be when research concerns ill or otherwise disadvantaged individuals. Graduate student Jude Drapeau and I carried out the interviews that could be arranged.

12. In addition to changing the names, I have masculinized any female pronouns in the homosexually-partnered woman's statements in order to protect her anonymity.

13. One of these men recently died of AIDS; the other refuses to be tested.

14. This was said by Ron, who decided that, although seropositive, his partner had not actually infected him with HIV but that instead he had picked the virus up on his own.

15. I can give no details without breaking my confidentiality and anonymity promise.

16. In the second group, Ron made an almost verbatim statement.

17. Most talk of this strategy concerned casual sexual liaisons, but Maria also discussed non-disclosure conjoined with protective action in relation to her now-defunct IDU practice. She said, "I had already been positive when I got into the drug scene and [I was trying to not be] sharing needles and I used [the excuse] — I never said that I was HIV positive. The deal with it was I used, 'I'm a hemophiliac' — and then I found out you can't catch nothing from that! [laughter] And then I went through that I had hepatitis, and that, 'You will get sick from it [so] I don't share needles.' But I would not say I was HIV positive — I didn't want anybody to know. And this one guy insisted on taking my needle — insisting! I mean, he was ready to beat me up for this thing! Fine; good [sarcastically; i.e., how stupid]. And a long, long time I stood on that [excuse]. I never told him; I never told him [the truth]. But I also did tell him that he could get something. He still insisted on taking that syringe."

18. At one point Eric also said, "Positive people shouldn't have sex with anyone."

19. However, some of the participants' comments made regarding condom symbolism, a few examples of which come later in the text, indicate some understanding of denial's psychocultural motivations.

20. Here I must note that participants probably represent those HIV-positive people who are actually *most* likely to use counseling services. They were listed on agency rosters, for one thing, indicating at least some interest in using public services; for another, they were comfortable enough with their seropositive status to come forward as participants (see also note 10). That even they did not use available counseling services is telling.

21. According to local agency staff members, the number of AIDS cases for the area is actually inflated, because it includes people who come home to die.

22. As shown in Chapter 3, whole groups are faulted by others for originating

the pandemic. Some blame Africans or Haitians, while others blame the CIA or white supremacists for the "AIDS Conspiracy" (Dalton 1989; Farmer 1992; Quimby 1992; Sobo 1993b; Turner 1993). Malicious non-disclosure by an individual differs little from a conspiratorial plot except that an individual rather than highly organized group lies lurking, ready to entrap.

23. Where many homosexual and bisexual men are served, offices and their staff should display gay-friendly attitudes, as by keeping up-to-date gay publications in waiting rooms.

Chapter 10
Circumventing Denial

Neither the Midwesterners that Chapters 5–8 were expressly concerned with nor the Southwesterners who spoke through Chapter 9 thought that AIDS would affect them. But denial alone cannot hold HIV and AIDS at bay; indeed, denial sometimes acts as a catalyst that enables HIV to spread because denial keeps people from acting to reduce their risk for infection. In light of this, a keen understanding of the mechanisms underlying denial is essential, and this book has been expressly concerned with exposing and describing them to that end.

AIDS-risk denial in the United States is tied to monogamy ideals and so to women's position in society and in relation to men. The poor urban Black women who participated in the study that is the crux of this book idealize monogamy and hope for loyal conjugal partners. For convenience, I have referred to all talk that describes this mainstream dream of fidelity, puts forth a claim of having achieved it, or supports a belief in its reality as the "Monogamy Narrative." The defensive strategy of making claims regarding one's own ability to correctly evaluate the sexual (and IV drug) history and so, supposedly, the HIV status of potential sexual partners is termed the "Wisdom Narrative."

While the Wisdom Narratives of uninvolved women who engage in casual sex as they search for suitable partners focus on their own prudence regarding men, women with steady partners embed talk of wise partner choices in Monogamy Narratives. They boast of having perfect, intact conjugal unions. They claim that condomless sex is only risky for other women, who must contend with disrespectful, cheating spouses. In making such claims, women embrace one of the most counterproductive aspects of most AIDS education messages: the erroneous advice that multiple partnering is the major AIDS-risk behavior (see Bolton 1992). Research reviewed by Margaret Nichols (1990) shows no correlation between seroconversion and the number of sexual partners a woman has.

In fact, it is not how many partners one has but what actions one participates in with them that affects one's risk for AIDS. Most women who get AIDS are infected not by one-night stands but by long-term partners with whom they have condomless sex (Reiss, 1991, as cited in Bolton 1992).[1]

This research focused on identifying the mechanisms underlying AIDS risk denial. In doing so it showed that, in addition to perpetuating stereotypes, simple materialist models of Black female sexuality ignore the enormous impacts that culturally conditioned social and emotional factors have on women's sex lives.[2] The research revealed much about heterosexual relationships and about risk perception; it documented and described many previously hidden aspects of poor Black women's lives; it expanded our understanding of aspects that other research had begun to explore. Furthermore, it described the experiences of a small group of HIV-positive individuals in relation to partnerships and sexual activity. Interestingly, denial among the (theoretically) seronegative may be confronted quite frequently by seropositive people seeking sexual partnership.

factors that do affect behavior.

The findings are certainly important theoretically and ethnographically, but they must not remain hidden in the ivory tower. An anthropological understanding of the factors that encourage unsafe sex can put health educators in a better position from which to combat them, for, as Bolton and Singer point out, "HIV prevention is first and foremost a problem in culture change" (1992, 2). And just as promoting or emphasizing certain cultural factors (e.g., the monogamy ideal) in AIDS education curricula discourages change, emphasizing select others can facilitate it.

"Sensitivity" may make educ. more effective

Research has shown that building cultural awareness and gender sensitivity into AIDS education and intervention programs can make them more effective (e.g., Amass et al. 1993; Bletzer 1993; Dorfman et al. 1992; Quirk 1993; Weeks et al. 1993; cf. Bolton and Singer 1992; Carovano 1991; Flaskerud and Rush 1989; Herdt and Boxer 1991; Leap and O'Connor 1993). The self-disclosure findings have been presented to AIDS service organizations in Las Cruces. Findings from the Cleveland study have been submitted for use by Dr. Toltzis and staff as they work to improve the M&I AIDS curriculum. These findings also might be incorporated into other programs designed to increase safer sex (and voluntary HIV-testing rates) within similar populations. They might be used to plan alterations of current AIDS education standards as well as of HIV-testing guidelines, counseling post-test, and condom distribution services so that they are more consistent with women's real needs. In this chapter, I suggest some of the directions that such alterations might take.

Education and Change

Standard Curricula Promote Unsafe Sex

In the previous chapters, I showed that the condom-related thoughts of the inner-city women who use Cleveland's M&I health services focus on the implications that condoms ("safeties") have regarding the relationships in which they are used. Condom use implicates one or both partners as unfaithful and infected, contradicting and undermining the Monogamy Narratives and Wisdom Narratives that women tell themselves and each other, forcing the personal acknowledgment of what women would deny: that relationships are not forever true.

Standard AIDS education curricula unintentionally promote unsafe sex rather than dissuade women from it because they make "wise" partner selection and monogamy seem like good alternates to condom use. The negative connotations that condoms have in regard to a relationship's quality are thereby reinforced. Further, condom use is often portrayed by educators as inconvenient and vexatious. In order for the pro-condom message to be heard, educators must change their own conceptions about condoms and alter their methods of promoting them; they also must change the attitudes they hold in regard to clinic clients and monogamy itself.

The following incident, which occurred during the education session held for one of the first-phase focus groups Margaret Ruble had been observing, reveals much in regard to women's feelings about philandering and the problems these beliefs pose for their personalization or internalization of AIDS risk information. It also bears witness to the attitudes some educators hold (even if unconsciously) toward clients.

The educator, a white woman, was discussing HIV tests. She had already told the women present that condoms must always be used, even between steady partners, because partners often cheat. She described the seropositivity lag: the window of time between initial infection and positive HIV status that makes it imperative for a monogamous couple to use condoms for several months after an HIV test and then get tested again before switching to condomless sex. She reminded the women that only the most committed couples could reach this point of condomless intimacy.

The educator then announced that she was engaged. She told the women that she and her future husband had been tested for HIV antibodies and that both of them were seronegative. She exclaimed how happy she was that she would never again have to worry about using condoms, which interrupt love-making and can be burdensome. Without realizing it, the educator had told the women that condoms were a bother and, more important, that she was different from them as her man would not cheat.

One might assume that the educator's double standard caused anger and frustration among the women. However, despite the implicit racism and classism, participants identified with the educator herself; they cast their own unions as similarly hermetically sealed or impervious and monogamous, following the Monogamy Narrative (cf. Kinsey 1994).[3] The educator's own denial of risk, clearly demonstrated in her statement about her future sexual practices, encouraged denial in many of the women being "educated" and reinforced their preconceived notion that there is no need for safer-sex within a faithful conjugal unit. And unsafe sex within a so-called faithful union helps a woman to maintain her state of denial and her belief that her partnership is one of love, trust, and fidelity. That even the AIDS educator told a Monogamy Narrative supports my contention that the denial processes I describe are pervasive among all women who buy into the monogamy ideal—not just among poor urban Blacks.

either combat the ideal or dissociate condoms from cheating (Δ meanings)

Alternative Approaches to AIDS Education

In the introduction to their collection of essays on AIDS prevention, Bolton and Singer write:

Prevention works best when it promotes change through individual and community empowerment strategies informed by holistic understandings of the local context, when it acknowledges the positive contributions of local cultural values to the process of change, and when it incorporates an array of options that permit individuals to transform their lives in ways that enhance their physical, emotional, and material well-being. Prevention efforts fail when they revictimize and stigmatize those who do not accept messages incompatible with their basic values and needs, when they blame those whose behavior suggests recalcitrance or relapse from risk standards established by health "experts," when they are based on top-down rather than community designed and implemented approaches, and when they are shaped by the moralistic and authoritarian models advocated by political, religious, and medical leaders whose agendas may be inimical to the best interests of the clients of many prevention programs. (1992, 4; italics in original)

Chapter 3 discussed the importance of maintaining sensitivity to local cultural values; here I shall suggest a number of ways this can be done in the inner city (these suggestions also can be adapted for use in other contexts where women subscribe to the monogamy ideal). To begin with, where self-determination is valued (as it is among many groups in the United States), educators must offer an array of options to each client (e.g., condoms plus other alternatives); this allows the client to maintain a sense of autonomy while diffusing negative attitudes about being told what to do (Taylor and Lourea 1992). In addition to describing varied safer-sex options, Bolton and Singer (1992) argue that interventions themselves should be varied. The more kinds of interventions offered in a given community (street outreach, clinic counseling, community center meetings, etc.) — and the more involved community members are in shaping these interventions — the more chance of success AIDS educators will have (regarding community-based intervention, see also Van Vugt 1994).

The blame and stigma that have been heaped on inner-city women for not using condoms stems from a reliance on (inappropriate) rational-action models as described in Chapter 3, and on (failed) "top-down" intervention planning that does not take real-life situations into account. The failure of those interventions stems in part from the moralistic appeal to monogamy that has infused AIDS education messages. Approaches to AIDS education that both glorify monogamy and offer condoms to non-monogamous ("bad") people undermine themselves because optimistic biasing leads most clients to cast themselves as monogamous ("good") people and so as being in no need of protection (cf. Bolton 1992), as was the case with those "educated" by the engaged AIDS educator, above.

Furthermore, because U.S. cultural understandings about AIDS itself involve negative moralistic connotations that, if personalized or applied to oneself, would lead to humiliation and a loss of self-esteem, even approaches that attempt to alter behavior by appealing directly to logic and risk calculations will fail; again, optimistic biasing (described in Chapter 3) will lead to risk misperception. This was the case not only with the majority of the Cleveland participants but also with many of the sex partners the seropositive Southwesterners described in the preceding chapter. Clearly, seropositive individuals need to be made aware by clinicians or counselors that optimism and AIDS-risk denial in sex partners is a cognitive artifact that must (for the sake of their own health) be countered by the seropositive with an insistence on prophylaxis rather than with an acceptance of partners' preference for condomless sex as if this was a fully informed personal choice.

In order to encourage rather than discourage women from practicing safer sex, educators need to recognize the particular cultural ideals and aspects of women's feelings about condoms, relationships, and men that can be productively appealed to (and which were described in the last few chapters). While the monogamy ideal is, overall and in itself, the wrong ideal to appeal to, certain aspects of cultural beliefs about ideal relationships can perhaps be advantageously exploited.

Capitalizing on the Concept of Care and on the Notion of Pleasure

Interviewee testimony showed that people often act wisely to protect their primary or inside partners if they are having sex with outside partners. One clinic focus group participant said in relation to an outside affair, "I play it wise," adding, "I always protect him and he goes for protection." For most women, however, protecting inside partners through condom use in the context of inside sexual action is, when viewed in light of accepted monogamy ideals, not an option. But if monogamy ideals are not brought to attention in interventions, women may more easily bypass the cognitive and emotional dissonance condom use would otherwise entail.

Condoms could be represented as symbolic of the true and loving relationships that many women strive for rather than as necessary armor to protect against partners who will surely cheat. Instead of challenging women's Monogamy and Wisdom Narratives by stressing the pervasiveness of multiple partnering or adultery, or insulting women by maligning their abilities to discriminate among men, educators might highlight the fact that even people who are faithful may carry HIV unawares. That is, a man may love a woman and refrain from having affairs and still he may have the virus (as may a woman). Condom use is then an act of altruistic love and commitment rather than an identity threatening admission of current philandering (cf. Kline et al. 1992). It shows that partners love one another, and it shows also that individuals love and respect themselves — which they easily can do without hating or fearing their lovers. Clinic interviewee Shelly loved her partner dearly and trusted him. Still, she insisted on condoms because, as she unhesitatingly proclaimed, "I love myself."

Self-love and love of others should be highlighted, and the link between knowledgeable altruism and risk reduction could be taken advantage of by those who would promote condom use among primary partners. Clinic interviewee Mary commented that she would tell future partners, "We want to protect each other." The wisdom of benevolent prophylaxis is particularly apparent to seropositive individuals (Chapter 9), and to mothers (Mays and Cochran 1988; Tunstall et al. 1991; Vander Linden 1993; Ward 1993a). The wisdom of altruistically protecting one's inside partner both directly through condom use and indirectly through condom use with outside lovers seems worth promoting in tandem with the notion of love. Here I should note that loving altruism is not a characteristic confined to women: the findings of Solomon and DeJong (1989) regarding the use of videotapes for condom promotion suggest that promotions for men will be more successful if they "portray clearly the health risks that unprotected intercourse creates for women and children" (457; regarding altruism see also Turner et al. 1989, 279). If a spouse's or child's health already has been affected, grief may provide motivation to reduce risk-taking behavior if sensitive intervention is provided (Nyamathi et al. 1990).

It is not enough to sell condoms as symbols of love and care when the loving, caring act of condom use is still presented or perceived of as a bother and a chore. In addition to the way that the above-featured AIDS educator's approach encouraged AIDS-risk denial, it inadvertently encouraged women to hold onto (or, in some cases, to develop) anti-condom sentiments by sending messages about how disruptive and bothersome condom use is. Participants throughout this research often associated condoms with discomfort and deadened sensation.

Men, especially, were said by the participants to gain more enjoyment when they could "feel the flesh" directly. Interviewee Nicole suggested that women who made men use condoms despite men's appeals for sensation acted unkindly. Interestingly, men are not the only ones with complaints about condoms. One-fourth of the forty-three Cleveland women who were interviewed over the course of the study (25.6%, n = 11)[4] reported that condoms interfered physically in their own sexual pleasure. As clinic focus group participants said in relation to the physical sensation of condom use, "It feels like a balloon to me," "It don't feel right period," "I can't say I had feeling with [condoms] once," "Without it, it feels better," and "I just prefer to have flesh."

My first inclination was to cast this kind of talk as rationalization: I thought that perhaps women who were coerced into condomless sex might seek to justify their behavior by saying that condoms do not feel nice anyhow. But details provided by participants as well as data from other studies confirm that condom use is a skill that is learned; without good skills, condoms can be problematic and even ineffective (Steiner et al. 1993; Thompson et al. 1993; cf. Kline et al. 1992). Further, without lubricant — and many of the condoms that clinics provide for free are dry — sex with condoms can be quite painful for receptors. More information on condom-related sexual skills and messages that encourage people to associate safer sex with pleasurable sex should be provided.

Positive information on how condoms can enhance sex (e.g., by helping men maintain their erections longer, by containing semen that might otherwise wet the bedsheets) and instruction on how to incorporate condoms into the sex act pleasurably could be a regular part of AIDS interventions. Tanner and Pollack (1988) found that couples who received eroticized instructions on condom use had significantly enhanced attitudes toward condoms (see also Jemmott and Jemmott 1991).[5] The sex-positive approach worked for the focus group participant who told her partner that "the rubbers will make him last longer."

In addition to condoms, the promotion of which suggests that penetrative-receptive intercourse involving the penis is the only legitimate form of sex, alternative safer-sex strategies should be promoted. Although Black women have, historically, had narrow sexual repertoires, this seems to be changing (see Chapter 2) and in the right context instruction on sexual techniques might be welcome. As Taylor and Lourea contend, "It is much easier for people to increase sexual options than to extinguish established patterns" (1992, 107).

knowledge can add but less effective e erasing

Group Interventions

Usually, M&I clinic education took place in one-on-one sessions. Questions a woman might not be able to raise in front of a group can be raised in such a context. But the quality of the discussion-group interactions and data from the interviews indicate that women should also meet in groups (cf. Shervington 1993). Participants said that they do not usually discuss HIV and AIDS in daily life; they welcomed the opportunity we provided to discuss what they see as a serious matter, and they told us that they generally enjoyed the experience. Indeed, in recent years there has been a trend toward group interventions in which "the women help one another by sharing information (on how they are coping with overwhelming multiple problems) and emotional support as the basis for individual attempts at behavior modification" such as attempting condom use (Worth 1989, 299; parentheses in original). It is reported that "there is a strong sense of mutual support among women [who participate in] intervention groups," and that "as the women develop rapport among themselves, they encourage each other to try out behavior changes" (Vander Linden 1993, 413).

Women who want to participate in such groups may feel embarrassed to ask clinic staff about meeting locations. Program coordinators can counter this by posting signs on clinic walls directing women to the proper rooms (Worth 1989). Program coordinators also can identify and use multiple alternative sites. This is necessary because many public health offices are uncomfortably furnished and institutional; furthermore, clinic procedures usually implicitly (and sometimes explicitly) encourage women to leave directly after being served. Cleveland participants frequented public libraries, beauty salons, and churches, and these settings—already seen by the women as comfortable places in which to pursue their own mental, physical, and spiritual development—could be used more frequently as AIDS education sites.

the location/PLACE of info presentation matters.

Women's homes also can be used: Planned Parenthood has initiated safer sex party programs in numerous low-income neighborhoods and reports good success (Stepp 1994). The parties generally involve a discus-

sion about sex, an AIDS videotape, a demonstration of how to put a
condom on a man's penis, and the distribution of pamphlets and condoms. In light of the fact that Black women (and men) give high cre-
dence to word of mouth (Mays 1989), such parties promise to be successful in spreading the pro-condom message.

While individual counseling should of course continue, it seems that
interventions offered in supportive group contexts can help women
build their sense of self-efficacy or self-assuredness and develop the coping skills necessary for putting aside the practice of unsafe sex (see Turner et al. 1989, 278–279 regarding empowering self-efficacy and social
skills training). Clinicians could purposefully attempt to exploit the band-
wagon effect in group session settings so that group interaction releases
women from believing that they are alone in wanting to use condoms (cf.
Valdiserri et al. 1989). Safer sex could be presented as the new norm
rather than as a bother and an exception (this should be done in the
popular media, too; cf. Fisher 1988).

Dealing with Misgivings and Misconceptions

Group meetings might also provide a setting conducive to combating
AIDS-related conspiratorial thought. Such thought releases people from
culpability but lends no support to safer-sex practices because infection
can come at any time and in any way. If AIDS interventions are to be
successful, they must provide people tools with which to manage this kind
of thinking. Focused group discussions might provide women with an
arena in which to air any conspiratorial thoughts. Importantly, as Thomas
and Quinn (1991) suggest, educators should allow clients plenty of room
to discuss their fears of genocide, and only after doing so should they
gently proceed to disabuse the women of these fears. That is, conspiracy
rhetoric cannot be simply dismissed out of hand. To do so would validate
clients' beliefs that the health care system does not care about them and
cannot be trusted (cf. DeParle 1990; Herek and Capitanio 1994).

AIDS educators must acknowledge that the racist abuse underlying
conspiracy fears does occur in the health-care system and they must allow
and help clients to work these experiences through. Second-phase interviewee Donna, a thirty-four-year-old mother of six, told me a disturbing
story in the context of a question regarding birth control that bears
repeating:

I have that shot, Depo Provera, right? I got upset when they gave me that shot
'cause . . . they just popped me up with this shot, right? And [only] a week later,
it was all in the news about them giving those shots to women in India and Africa, and in the United States it's not even [accepted] — I thought that was so
wrong. . . . And they did it while I was breast-feeding. They told me my baby

would not get that, and, and I just thought it was wrong. How could they do that? I thought because I was Black, that they did that to me. [Without asking permission, the nurse] came in and stuck me with that. . . . She was like, "Here, you won't get pregnant now."

people have good reason to distrust certain sources of knowledge

Because such abuses do occur, AIDS educators need to show that they have clients' best interests at heart. Those who come from the communities served may be able to convey such a message most credibly.

Beyond restoring or raising clients' faith in the health care system, educators also need to debunk the typical misconceptions that linger long after clients' factual knowledge regarding AIDS has been increased. This might best be done not through labeling such beliefs as "superstition" and then dismissing them but rather by offering common-sense explanations as to why they are in error. For example, it makes sense to think that mosquitoes can transmit AIDS until one learns about the environments in which the virus can and cannot survive. The fact that AIDS is not endemic in swampy areas where mosquitoes thrive also can be used to calm mosquito-related AIDS fears. Common-sense beliefs must be fought with common-sense logic.

Another thought problem that educators should address has to do with cognitive processes rather than cognitive content. I already have discussed (and suggested ways to avert) women's use of unsafe sex to avoid the dissonance that condom use in primary relationships can otherwise create as it brings together ideas better kept apart: monogamy ideals and thoughts of infidelity. Here, I draw attention to another potentially dissonant experience resolved through condomless sex. In addition to infection prevention, condoms also can prevent conception, and so using them when one has had a tubal ligation or uses another family planning method can seem redundant. Focus group participants said that when asked to use condoms men generally respond coercively: "Baby, don't you take birth control?" If the answer is yes (or if the woman has an IUD, etc.), that generally settles the issue. A cognitive shift takes place, and the original prophylactic intent of condom use is forgotten. AIDS educators need to increase people's awareness of the probability that they may fall prey to this common error.

Adversarial or Complementary Conjugal Relations and Prophylactic Technologies

Importantly, in all their endeavors educators must avoid trying to set women against men, which they do when casting all men as evil philanderers who need to be stood up to (and which they would probably never do in appeals to middle-class whites).[6] Such tactics for empowerment will backfire because, rather than focusing on the culturally idealized complementary dimensions of relationships, they cast relationships as adversarial. Adversarial models of conjugality do not make sense to women as they consider their own sexual relations, for such models contradict the idealized complementary models women strive to actualize with their partners. Presenting condoms as symbolic of conjugal love rather than as needed protection against deceitful men is one way around the potential pitfall of making inappropriate intimations about women's relationships.[7]

Up until now, I have not discussed the female condom. This is mostly because the apparatus — a tubular plastic-bag-like sheath with a firm ring lining its flared opening, and which anchors itself outside of the vagina by means of this ring — was not available when the research was carried out, nor is it easily available as I write this chapter. However, as it has been optimistically hailed as a device that puts women in control of STD and AIDS prevention by some clinicians, some women's health advocates, and even by some women who would use it (but who have not yet done so; e.g., Shervington 1993), the female condom deserves mention here.

I fear that the female condom may fail to fulfill expectations. Its concealed use for self-protective STD and AIDS prevention suggests an adversarial model of conjugality, which many women will find offensive. And secrecy will be impossible anyhow: given the condom's large outer ring, men will notice it. I believe that they will react much as they might react to condoms. Furthermore, data from focus groups of impoverished Black women show that they would actually expect their men to be involved in the device's use (Shervington 1993); this attitude is quite distinct from the one involving cunning secret control that many clinicians promoting female condoms talk about. In fact, it supports the complementary rather than the adversarial model of conjugality.

While the female condom may not turn out to be the AIDS panacea once thought, there is at least one other female-controllable AIDS protection device on the horizon. The World Health Organization seeks to develop a safe, effective microbicide that can be inserted into the vagina. Ideally, it would not bother microbes that exist naturally in the vagina and promote health. Also, it would not impair women's ability to have children by harming sperm or by altering the vaginal environment, as many women have no interest in contraception or have spouses against contraception (Altman 1993). In any case, such a product could easily be used without male knowledge and so would relieve women from their dependence on men for prophylactic cooperation. When and if this microbicide is developed — provided that it is promoted not by talk of philandering boyfriends and husbands but rather by appeals to women's

ideas about personal health and hygiene, self-determination, and altruistic love (much as birth control pills are) — it promises to be widely
accepted.

Appealing to Men

To whom is the info targeted?

The emphasis on vaginal microbicides and female condoms parallels, in
some ways, sexist family planning research trends, in which women's and
not men's bodies are seen as appropriate sites for contraceptive intervention. In discussing vaginal microbicides, female condoms, and women's
need to persuade their male partners to use penile condoms, I do not
mean to reproduce this bias by implying that women should bear the sole
responsibility for HIV-transmission prevention. Men should, without fail,
take part in prophylactic efforts. However, as with contraception, women
must watch out for themselves; for sociocultural reasons already discussed, they cannot at present rely on male participation.

While ways can be suggested for AIDS educators to help women improve their condom use rates (including advice on how to persuade men
to see that condoms are good things), educational interventions aimed
directly at improving men's condom-related attitudes would make wom-
en's task here much easier. Heterosexual penetrative-receptive intercourse generally involves two bodies, and so two wills. These wills, male
and female, gain their expression in particular social and cultural contexts. The context of inner-city women's sex lives has already been detailed. Because men are in many ways the leading players in that sexual
arena because of women's emotional and social dependence on them;
interventions directed toward men are essential.

Historically, most AIDS interventions (with the exception of those
geared toward injecting drug users) have targeted women, not only because of concern for their potential progeny, but also (and, in terms
of logistics, more importantly) because women's reproductive health
needs bring them into clinics much more frequently than men, making
them a kind of captive audience. This female bias needs to be corrected
for.

I cannot, on the basis of this research, offer empirically-based recommendations regarding male-directed AIDS interventions. But some suggestions can be made. First, increasing the number of male-directed condom ads would help convince men to do their part (currently, most ads
target women [Muir 1991, 154]). These ads might appeal specifically to
the inner-city male's focus on hyper-masculine behavior, presenting condoms as symbols of virility or as manly in themselves. Ads also might take
advantage of the fact that many economically and socially disadvantaged

inner-city men rely heavily on peer evaluation as a source of self-esteem (Anderson 1990; Liebow 1967).

Because of this reliance on peer evaluation, group-centered education programs might help to shift men's condom-related attitudes and practices.[8] The unbalanced relationship between power and gender makes such a shift crucial if women's decisions to use condoms are to be implemented. To this end, some of these groups might be mixed. I mentioned that men shown videotapes concerning women's and children's risks for HIV infection were motivated to reduce their risks (Solomon and DeJong 1989). Exposing men to women directly, in the context of a group intervention, could also encourage risk reduction action.

Mixed gender groups could lead to better inter-gender understandings and so help to clear up misconceptions that the genders have about each other. For example, men might not actually have such negative views about condoms as women think they do (cf. Kegeles et al. 1988; Schoenborn et al. 1994). If women learn from men that this is true, they may be more interested in suggesting condom use. Without our asking about it, the women in this research expressed interest in learning more about men's thoughts regarding sex and AIDS. Clinic focus group participants directly requested that the moderator bring men into the project. Further, they responded to some issues with statements such as, "I would love to hear [the men's] answer to that."

Improving HIV Test Uptake Rates

Making condoms seem part of a standard accepted routine promises to increase condom use rates as people who buy into mainstream values strive to fit in socially. Findings suggest that the same tactic will work with HIV antibody testing. Chapter 8 showed that health center clients prefer to think of HIV tests as routine, particularly when speaking face-to-face with other women. Clinicians must respect this. When clinicians cast HIV tests as commonplace and customary rather than as necessitated by social and moral breeches (such as infidelity) the tests become less emotionally (and socially) threatening to clients. Women will be much more likely to agree to a routine procedure than they will to a test that undermines their faith in their own conjugal relations (or that promises benefits they know cannot currently be delivered). As with condoms, which people might use more often if cast as symbolic of nurturance, cooperation, love, and respect rather than disease and betrayal (see Chapter 7; cf. Boyd 1990; De Bruyn 1992; Mays and Cochran 1988), test-taking should be motivated not by messages meant to increase perceived susceptibility, but by those that appeal to normative cultural values and that enhance self-esteem, thereby making each action a logical as well as a prudent choice.

Education and Employment

While improved interventions will help increase condom use rates, they are not the whole answer. Inner-city women and men also need improved educational and employment opportunities. Study findings indicate that jobs outside the home can provide women with at least some of the self-esteem and status for which too many now rely solely on men. As Anitra Pivnick suggests, employment can "generate feelings of accomplishment, independence, and personal worth" (1993, 449). Such feelings can enhance women's ability to insist on condoms as these feelings reduce women's emotional and social dependence on men. And were more jobs available for inner-city men, they would not need to base their manhood so heavily on fathering children, keeping multiple sexual partners, and asserting dominance within the sexual arena.

Concluding Remarks

Women's Current Position on Condom Use and AIDS

The following excerpt comes from an interview with Nicole, who was twenty years of age when we spoke, and very pregnant. A gregarious, sociable young woman, Nicole dressed in the latest fashion and planned to go into cosmetology. Like the other women, Nicole felt that condoms are for extraconjugal sexual liaisons only. To introduce them in a primary relationship signals problems.

As we were about to end the interview, I asked Nicole if she felt that I had forgotten to ask about anything that might be important in relation to male-female relationships, sexuality, or AIDS, or if she had anything to add. She began to talk about her own relationship:

That's my man: that's my favorite partner, and I'm having sex with him. He should be having sex with [only] me. If he's having sex with somebody else, and brings home AIDS, and I die from AIDS, you know, that just really will have to happen, because I'm not going to worry about a condom. I can't worry about if he was having sex and bringing me home [diseases]. But if I did get AIDS and he gave it to me and—I would kill him flat out. So we're going to be together either way it go. I mean, it's just something that—I feel that—I mean everybody is stressing [AIDS], and you know, OK, we have to work harder, but I've [only] been to bed with maybe three guys in my entire life, you know. If I got AIDS, then you know, I just got AIDS and I'm gonna die from it and that's just it. It's a big deal, it really is, and I know it is, but I'm not [going to] walk around here like a hypochondriac worrying about AIDS. I don't shoot up; I'm not gay and my boyfriend isn't gay. What I'm saying [is] I don't abuse, I don't go to the hospital and just get blood drawn and give it, so I'm not a high risk. If I get AIDS [it's because] God knows that's what I needed and He's killing me off, you know, because—He has my best interests at hand anyway. I'm not worried about AIDS; I really don't worry about AIDS. And it's like it's a shame, 'cause maybe I should.

Nicole's response contains illustrations of several dimensions of AIDS risk perception, and in its progression it demonstrates the switchbacks or cognitive spirals I think we all engage in when thinking about our own risks for AIDS. The discourse moves from talk about how Nicole's partner would neither cheat nor bring home AIDS to talk about what she would do if he did. Her proposed response reveals anger and dismay even while it demonstrates her dependence on and commitment to her man ("we're going to be together either way it go"). This kind of commitment or love is one of the reasons individuals in relationships with seropositive people, such as Maria's partner (Chapter 9), sometimes refuse to use condoms: they have no interest in living without their partners (Pivnick 1993).

Like most women, Nicole agrees that AIDS is a pervasive, frightening problem. She admits in the context of the interview that her partner, like any man, may be cheating. But she cannot worry about this, because unfaithfulness is not really expected. Nor is it condoned. If it did happen, her partner's infidelity would be just cause for anger. Moreover, it would undermine the model Nicole presents of her relationship—a model just like the basic relationship model most mainstream Americans aspire to and would present. In any case, Nicole cannot be bothered with condoms. The optimistic bias underlies her feeling that none of her behavior puts her at risk: she does not shoot up, sleep around, or have sex with a man who (to her knowledge) has sex with men or with other women. Like many inner-city women, she probably also has other immediate risks to deal with regularly, like neighborhood crime and her pregnancy. She may have neither time nor energy left to worry about AIDS.

While certainly not all women would have referred to God's will when discussing their possible contraction of AIDS, the kind of attributional or extrapunitive thought that Nicole's assignment of responsibility to God demonstrates was typical among most women. That is, optimistic biases and mistaken beliefs about AIDS transmission led most women to believe that if they did "catch AIDS" it would not be because of something that they themselves did. They felt that although they did what they could to lower their risks (using condoms for extraconjugal sex, choosing partners wisely, staying away from injection drugs, etc.) they had little control over their own possible infections because they might be infected through tainted transfusions, vindictive individuals, or even (although in their eyes the probability was not likely) by lying, cheating spouses.

Study Conclusions

The psychosocial strategy of having unsafe sex leaves intact rosy façades and culturally engendered dreams of monogamy, security, and white picket fences. In some senses then unsafe sex is an adaptive and defensive practice. It helps women maintain desired, idealized images of partners, relationships, and selves, and these are mainstream American as well as Black inner-city images. But the long-term costs of unsafe sex can be devastating, especially when practiced in the context of poverty, racism, and sexism. Accordingly, women must forsake it.

The research findings suggest that reducing women's dependence on men and increasing their access to alternative sources of self-esteem and social status would hasten changes in sexual practice. But the AIDS pandemic will not wait for us to restructure race, power, and gender relations. The simplest, quickest way to increase safer sex rates among impoverished urban minority women — the women most vulnerable to infection — involves adjusting AIDS education curricula so that they give women and their present social and emotional needs the respect they are due.

Notes

1. Multiple partnering may, however, increase a woman's risk for other sexually transmitted diseases and thereby render her more vulnerable to HIV transferred into her bloodstream during sex with her main partner (Nichols 1990).

2. A deeper analysis of the shortcomings of simple political economy models of HIV infection than this book was able to provide due to space limitations is found in Sobo (n.d.).

3. First-phase interviewees were asked whether it mattered that many of the scientists and professionals that promote safer sex are white. Only one woman said yes; the rest said that color made no difference. Three-quarters (77.8%, N = 18) were glad that AIDS educators of any racial or ethnic background took interest in them; one-third (27.8%) specifically mentioned that it was nice that people cared enough to warn them about risky behaviors. These views, and the fact that so many poor urban women aspire to careers in health, may make their identification with white AIDS educators easier.

4. This includes four women from the first phase (22.2%, N = 18) and seven from the second phase (28%, N = 25).

5. Tanner and Pollack (1988) recruited thirty-six heterosexual couples, ostensibly for a study of condom color preferences. The couples were divided into three groups, one receiving eroticized use instructions, the second receiving clinical use instructions, and the third receiving no instructions at all. Couples were provided colored condoms at random. They were asked to use six condoms in a two-week period, after which they completed a questionnaire and were debriefed.

6. Philip Toltzis first made this point explicit.

7. Cline et al. suggest that "individuals may take partners' willingness to talk about AIDS, in any fashion, as evidence of honesty and openness" (1990, 806), and so advising women that good communication with their partners about AIDS and condoms can enhance their relationships, perhaps bringing them even further in line with the idealized form, is another possible tactic. However, as Cline et al. warn, when people see honesty and openness in a partner they may cast that partner as being completely faithful or of "lesser risk" (806), which could lead them to forgo condoms unless popular ideas about monogamy are repudiated through AIDS education.

8. At least among one group of mostly Black adolescents, those who perceived peer norms as supportive of condom use were significantly more likely to use condoms consistently (DiClemente 1992). This is not to imply that men and adolescents are comparable but simply to suggest that the effects of peer condom-use norms on adults — especially those blocked from living up to adult role expectations — are worth investigating.

Appendix A: Interviewee Profiles

The following brief profiles include information on age, number of children, job status, conjugal status, contraception preferences, goals, and demeanor for each participant in the final (clinic) interview portion of the research. Any woman designated as a condom user reported using condoms during her last sexual encounter before being interviewed. With the exception of statements regarding dress and general demeanor, the information listed for each woman was provided by that woman. The descriptions are written in the ethnographic present.

Adrienne: Forty-five-year-old Adrienne has three children of her own and also cares for three grandchildren. She is very disapproving of men, partly because of the problems she has experienced with the father of her children, who provided no support, did not return her love, and was jealous and domineering. Adrienne has been with her current partner for only a month and in fact is not sure if she will stay with him (she said that she was involved when screened for the interview). She does not work but would like to go into nursing. She is presently enrolled in one of the parenting classes administered by the social welfare bureau, and in treatment for drug use. She cooks at the church on the days that they set up their soup kitchen. Adrienne has had a tubal ligation.

Bernice: Twenty-four-year-old Bernice, a condom user, has a five-year-old daughter. Bernice had recently served several months in prison. Her boyfriend moved on while she was incarcerated but she still loves him deeply. Bernice has a new boyfriend of three months who is good to her, and seems sweet (he is eager to use condoms to make her happy), but she cannot get over her former partner. She maintained a flat demeanor throughout the interview, suggesting that she was depressed. Still, despite her troubles Bernice is trying to improve her existence. She is enrolled in a life skills training program administered by the city's social welfare system and she would like to go to school to prepare for a job in hospitality or as a dietitian.

Betsy: Betsy is twenty-five years old and two months pregnant with a wanted child. She has been with — and been abused by — her partner for six years. The man drinks, and he is very jealous. She has left him several times but always ends up back with him. She knows she can go home to her family, but she does not do so. Betsy just took the high school equivalency test. She has a part-time cleaning job but she wants to be a nurse's assistant. She keeps no friends apart from her sisters. She never uses family planning methods.

Carol: Twenty-year-old Carol has her baby with her at the clinic. She is in college, engaged, and lives with her boyfriend of sixteen months. Carol acts quite mature. She used to be more proper, she says, but her boyfriend talked her into loosening up. Her concern with her demeanor comes from the fact that she always wants to make a good impression and worries about not doing her best. She is not only more relaxed now, she says, but also more social. Her boyfriend encourages that. He is not the jealous type. Carol has plans to be a lawyer or an accountant. She is a hard worker. She uses birth control pills and sometimes foam as well.

Clarissa: At twenty-eight, Clarissa has three children and a baby on the way. Her husband of ten years was just incarcerated for domestic violence (perpetrated against her). Still, she says that he loves her, and she feels that she cannot kick him out of her house as he has nowhere to go. She views him as one of her children although she wishes he would grow up (get a job, stop drinking, etc.). Clarissa does not like public places, as she suffers from anxiety attacks. She feels that she has no job skills. With birth of her third child, she realized she was "the man of the family" and decided to go back to school (she is interested in nursing). But she got pregnant, and her husband's abuse got worse. Clarissa does not keep many friends, and she is not cheerful. While she once used birth control pills, she does not use any family planning method regularly now.

Dee: At thirty-six, Dee has one child and has been with her partner for nineteen years. She does secretarial work. She and her partner lived together once, but they do not do so any longer. His little habits and his jealousy got on her nerves and she kicked him out. Dee has plans to go back to school and to study computer programming. She wants to stay with her present employer, but to move up to a better position. She has had an IUD for eighteen years.

Donna: Thirty-four-year-old Donna is a big, well-groomed woman with a handsome face. She has six children and is newly involved with a man she met five months ago. She is not sure where the relationship will go; she is feeling a bit crowded at the moment. Donna is not a very social person because so many of her friends got involved in the drug world — a world she wants no part of. Donna does hair for $85–$100 or more a head, and with three heads a week can make up to $400 or so weekly. Still, she would like to go into nursing. She has had her tubes tied and so does not use birth control.

Falasha: Serious, soft-spoken Falasha is very thin although she is pregnant. She is twenty-four years old and has an eight-year-old son. The baby she is expecting was sired by her boyfriend of four and one-half years. He is thirty-seven and steadily employed, as is she. Both are members of a religion that (among other things) promotes vegan diets and teaches that women are not men's equals. Falasha does not believe in birth control but, as she is pregnant, she and her boyfriend use condoms to protect the baby from his semen's toxicity (Falasha is considered a condom user). The couple plan on getting married. They share expenses but still keep separate bank accounts. Falasha does not socialize at work but has many friends in the church.

June: Thirty-five-year-old June, a tidy woman, is in treatment for substance use. She lives with her mother and has been with her primary partner for two years. She has been seeing a secondary beau for two weeks. She has not told her primary partner about her drug habit or about her outside man. She uses condoms for family planning. June emphasizes family and church in her responses. She lost her last formal job in 1989, and now sells flowers on street corners on holidays and helps with a grocery-store jitney (transport) service. June likes this work and she can make ten to twenty dollars a day helping out. But she has her AA and wants to continue her education. June speaks in measured sentences and circumlocutiously, using vague and erudite words. She does not maintain an active social life.

Linda: Twenty-four-year-old Linda does secretarial work. Her husband of four years is also employed. As he works a night shift, he cares for their two children during the day. Linda appears very middle class in dress, grooming, and language. She is very family oriented and does not keep many friends. She has plans, as does her husband, to return to school to finish an AA degree. She would like to go into nursing or perhaps social work. Linda has had her tubes tied.

Marvelle: At twenty-one, Marvelle is expecting her first child. A large woman, she is dressed for clinic in a new denim outfit heavily accessorized with gold jewelry. Marvelle's nails are painted and very long, and her hair is in a style that costs $45 a week to maintain. She is not employed. Marvelle was not practicing family planning, never thought she would get pregnant, and is not very happy about her condition. She also is not too happy with her boyfriend of one and one-half years (a drug dealer). He does not want to let her go to bars and parties but he goes out whenever he wants. They bicker frequently. Still, Marvelle loves him. He wants her to go to college and major in business. She might study history instead.

Mary: Thirty-six-year-old Mary, mother of one, is statuesque. She has her hair cropped close, and wears small gold hoop earrings, a denim shirt, and jeans. She is a smart, open, straight-talking woman. Mary is in treatment for drug use and currently stays with her mother, who handles all her finances. She has no job but does a little baby-sitting or cleaning for pay when she can. Mary does not keep friends except for Jesus. She thanks him for the fact that her boyfriend of ten years stayed with her even when she was deep into her drug habit. Mary does not practice birth control.

Michelle: Dressed in a new-looking outfit, her hair long and coifed and her long nails painted, nineteen-year-old Michelle has been in a relationship for two years. She emphasizes her beau's honesty and his willingness to do things for her. Michelle is an ex-cheerleader who got good grades; she does not drink or smoke and is not really very social. She lives with her mother. Her goal is to go into social work. Michelle never has sex without a condom (she is a condom user); she does not want to get pregnant.

Nicole: Nicole is a bubbly, sociable twenty-year-old. She is big and fashionable, with coifed hair and lots of make-up. She is interested in cosmetology. Unlike many of the interviewees, she appears fine financially. Nicole, who does not practice birth control, is pregnant with her first child. Her boyfriend of three years is in jail but will be out before her baby is born. He is excited about the pregnancy and Nicole says that he will put aside his wicked ways when he gets out of prison. He did deal in drugs and gave her lots of money ($2,000+ per mo.) which she missed at first but does not pine for anymore. She got herself a job as a nurse's aide and she feels good about that. When Nicole describes her boyfriend, she mentions the fact that he never hits her.

Pam: Pam is thirty-seven years old and a mother of two. She is small, and her hair is short and has been straightened. She is in treatment for drug use and in a sales management training program. Pam wears a blazer, skirt, and black blouse buttoned high. She is pragmatic and business-like but also fidgety and nervous; she asks me what I want her to say. She has been with her current partner for two years. She calls herself a loner and a manipulator. Pam does not practice birth control because she feels that when her time to bear comes, her time comes.

Peg: Thirty-four-year-old Peg has been in recovery for three weeks. She and her boyfriend of three-quarters of a year both lost their jobs one week ago, because of drugs. Peg's mother is a very influential figure in her life but also meddlesome (she drives Peg's friends away). Her mother calls Peg manipulative, and she allows that it is true: she only deals with people who can give her something. She will manipulate men but not with her body. Peg has one girlfriend from grade school but still keeps many secrets and is a private person. For family planning, she had a tubal ligation.

Penny: Twenty-two-year-old Penny has one son and is pregnant. She had been using birth control pills but "got careless," partly because her husband, whom she has known for seven years, was incarcerated until recently. She just left him, due to his crack addiction. Despite their being married, theirs was an on-again-off-again relationship. Her husband often saw other women. Even though her husband was possessive and jealous, she saw other men. Still, she did not really consider any of them as boyfriends. Men lie and cheat, she says; her husband has always let her down. Penny keeps few friends of either sex, and is in dire financial straits.

Roberta: Roberta is thirty-eight and although frazzled in appearance she is very thoughtful and deliberate when answering my questions and discussing her life. Her ultimate goal is to buy a house for herself and her son, but she does not have a job. She is looking for hospital work. Roberta has been with her current boyfriend for two years. He cheats but he "respects" her (i.e., he does not tell her about it). She cheated on him last year. She had a tubal ligation and does not like how condoms feel physically.

Rose: Thirty-six-year-old Rose, a mother of four, is a receptionist. She is well-groomed and an avid churchgoer. She does not keep many friends outside church, although she socializes on the job and likes to meet new people. Her vocation after work is sewing. Rose's boyfriend of five years lives with her; he has his own room. He works as a mechanic. He is extremely jealous. Rose had her tubes tied and does not use condoms.

Ruth: Twenty-five-year-old Ruth, a mother of one, has recently undergone major surgery. A condom user, she is friendly and wryly cynical. Her hair is a mess and she points to it when explaining that she generally is not bothered about careful grooming. Ruth is in love with her husband of six years but unsatisfied with the poor way he treats her. He drinks and acts irresponsibly; he did not support her through her surgery. Ruth is an avid churchgoer and sings in the choir. Most of her socializing revolves around the church. Her sister-in-law sits in on the interview, with her child; she prefers it this way and she says that the woman knows everything about her anyhow. For family planning purposes, Ruth gets injections of Depo Provera.

Sarah: Sarah is twenty-one; she has no children. Her boyfriend of two and one-half years would like her to have a baby for him and so they do not use contraception. The boyfriend is domineering. He wants her to wear fuller skirts, show less skin, and so forth. She baits him by telling him that he cannot tell her what to do until he marries her. She tells him that if he wants to leave her to go ahead; she is that sure of the relationship (although he did leave her once, and she cried and cried). At the same time, she feels old and she knows that it may be hard to find a new boyfriend. Sarah plans to be a nurse.

Shari: Twenty-seven-year-old Shari, a condom user who has one child, refuses to be taped but is talkative, and seems to sense that her words are important. On her own, she volunteers to talk slowly so that I can write down all she says, and she waits patiently if she sees that I am still writing. Shari works for her partner in his corner grocery shop. She is a certified nurse's aide. She thinks that she may go back to school. She uses condoms for birth control.

Shelly: Twenty-three-year-old Shelly, a mother of one, is in treatment for substance use. She was incarcerated on drugs and robbery charges for several years; she just got out and is on probation. She seems in a hurry. Shelly is sexually conservative and a condom user. She took things slow with her current boyfriend, whom she has known for a while but has only classed as boyfriend for four months, and she has never had sex without a condom (ever — her pregnancy was the result of a broken condom). She also uses foam. Shelly is not very social. In the future, she would like to get her high school equivalency diploma and become a nurse's aide.

Vicki: Vicki is a very mature nineteen years old. She has two children and one baby on the way. She is tidy for her clinic visit, dressed in shorts. Vicki does not drink or use drugs. She intends to go to nursing school. In the meantime, she has done some volunteer work at the library. She does not keep many friends; people can be too grudgeful. Vicki has been with her partner for five years. She keeps lovers on the side. While she does not practice family planning regularly, she does use condoms with these outside men.

Winsome: Thirty-four-year-old Winsome is a warm woman who wears her hair in a braid and is dressed in a modest sweater and jeans. She has nine children. For family planning purposes, she had a tubal ligation. Her boyfriend of six years is forty-seven. She has lived with him for three years and he supports her fully. She is now in treatment for drug use. Her beau makes her lunch, drops her off, picks her up, and even goes grocery shopping with her. She wants to work, but he will not let her. This caused their last fight, and they broke up for two or three months before getting back together.

Appendix B: Further Quantitative Findings

This appendix contains detailed quantitative data that complement findings already presented. The data, which are organized by subject matter, are not intended to stand on their own: the chapter of reference is noted after each subject heading.

1. Condom Use and Conjugal Status (Chapter 6)

Table B1 shows condom use (or non-use) at last sexual encounter by conjugal status for pilot questionnaire respondents. Interestingly, involved non-users had been involved with their partners for much longer than involved users had. Six of the twelve users were not involved at all. Four of the six involved users had been in their relationships for less than five years; two had been involved for five to nine years; none had been involved for over ten years. In contrast, seven of the fifteen involved non-users had been involved for more than five years; five of these seven — one-third of all fifteen — had been involved for over ten years.

2. Women's Income (Chapter 6)

Forty-four women provided explicit income information on the final questionnaire. The average total monthly income of condom users and non-users was essentially identical ($598.89 vs. $598.79). Nonetheless, when the averages from differing income sources are viewed in isolation, distinctions between the groups can be seen (see Table B2). (No significant differences in age, education, or number of children existed between the groups. Because of this, and because of the small sample size, such variables were not controlled for in statistical calculations. The figures given are merely descriptive.)

Users brought in smaller monthly paychecks than non-users. The average user's monthly pay was $147.80; the average non-user's was $252.93.

TABLE B1. Conjugal Status and Condom Use Among
Pilot Questionnaire Respondents

	Users (N=12)	Non-users (N=17)
Partnered	6	15
Single	6	2

TABLE B2. Women's Income Averages and Condom Use Patterns

Income source	Users (N=10)	Non-users (N=34)
Paid labor	$147.80	$252.93
Entrepreneurial schemes	0	$16.18
Assistance checks	$142.20	$145.65
Male partners	$308.89	$184.03
Total	$598.89	$598.79

Further, non-users generated additional income through entrepreneur-ial action while users did not. The average amount brought in through such efforts by non-users was $16.18; the average amount for users was nil. Assistance checks, however, were about the same size for members of either group: users received an average of $142.20; non-users $145.65.

After quantifying their incomes, respondents were asked if they relied on anyone at all to give them money regularly. Nine of the ten users and all thirty-four non-users provided at least one name. Thirty-two of the thirty-four non-users provided a second name as well. Although three spaces were provided, nobody named a third individual. While users gen-erally relied on one person and non-users generally relied on two, the average amount the named individuals contributed was similar: users re-ceived an average of $55.56, and non-users received an average of $56.06.

The purposefully open-ended nature of this question meant that women may have forgotten to list significant contributors. My particular interest was in how many women would mention men when asked indi-rectly as opposed to how many would mention them if asked directly. In the open-ended format, ten of the forty-four women listed partners as income sources. When asked directly, the number of women reporting income from men tripled. The income noted in response to the direct question was the figure used in the average monthly income calculations being described.

Here, I should note that when all questionnaire respondents are con-sidered (rather than just those for whom specific numerical financial data are available), a strikingly similar pattern is seen. Only eighteen (20%, N = 90) women named a partner as a source of aid in response to the open-ended question about support. But in response to the direct inquiry, fifty-five (61.1%) women affirmed that their partners sometimes gave them money; that is, thirty-seven more women (41.1%) remembered ever receiving cash from a partner. It is important to note that the group of thirty-seven additional women includes those who got only sporadic help. Moreover, thirty-five (38.9%) of the ninety women remained without men's monetary aid completely.

Of the forty-four sexually active women for whom I have specific financial data, thirty-two (72.7%) received some financial help from men. Twelve (27.3%) did not. The range of male contributions reported by the forty-four was the same for both condom-users and non-users: zero to $1,000. But users received an average of $308.89 from partners while non-users received an average of $184.03. The difference is $124.86. While users received, on average, significantly more male financial aid than non-users did, slightly more non-users received money at all: twenty-six (three-fourths) of the thirty-four non-users but only six (three fifths) of the ten users mentioned a male-provided income. (When average male-provided incomes are calculated for just those claiming them, the discrepancy grows. For the six users actually receiving male aid, male-provided income averages out to $463.34. For the twenty-six non-users, the average dollar amount is $219.42. The difference is $243.92.)

3. Condom Use Decisions (Chapter 6)

As seen in Chapter 6, just over half (55.6%) of the fifty-four final questionnaire respondents who provided information about both last condom use and condom use decision-making said that the decision to use or not use condoms is a joint one; just under half (42.6%) make the decision for themselves, by themselves. Similarly, as Table B3 shows, nine (50%) of the eighteen first-phase interviewees said that the decision to forgo condoms was arrived at through consensus. When those first-phase women who explained the decision as mutual after first claiming to have decided by themselves what to do about condoms are figured in, the number of dual decision-making women rises to twelve (66.7%). Seven (38.9%) of the eighteen women first spoke of the decision to skip condoms as entirely her own.

While focus group participants did hold that men often say no to condoms and almost eight in ten first-phase interviewees thought that the majority of men would not agree to use one when asked by a woman, in only two instances (11.1%) did interviewees' partners make the decision to leave the condoms off unilaterally. In one case (5.6%), the man originally agreed to use a condom but then "just shoved [his penis] in" unsheathed when sex began, leaving the woman quite angry and destroying the union. In the second case the woman "went along" to keep her man happy. Such deference represented only one in twenty (5.6%) cases.

TABLE B3. Condom Use Decision-Making Style for Phase-Two
Questionnaire Respondents and Phase-One Interviewees

	Questionnaire Respondents (N=54)	Interviewees (N=18)
Joint	30 (55.6%)	9 (50%)
Self-determined	23 (42.6%)	7 (38.9%)
Male-determined	1 (1.8%)	2 (11.1%)

Women who participated in the first phase of the research told us that male resistance to condoms and to female requests that they use them is omnipresent. Women may claim this to rationalize their own need for unsafe sexual contact and to mystify their responsibility for it. But if men do generally refuse condoms, as data so far indicate, many of the myriad reports of jointly decided upon condomlessness may represent strategic efforts to recast that which must be (i.e., unsafe sex) as that which is chosen. Calling the decision to forgo condoms "mutual" may reduce feelings of powerlessness. It also may camouflage emotional, social, and even economic dependence on men (however small — or large — the latter may be). This is not to say that real joint decision-making is an illusion or to imply that women never actually desire unsafe sex. Indeed, according to my denial hypothesis, women do want to have condomless intercourse; agreeing to unsafe sex reflects a real desire to signal commitment and repress knowledge of a relationship's fragility. I must acknowledge that if the desire is defensive it is in many ways not freely chosen; however, all choices are in some way constrained.

4. Non-Cash Contributions from Men (Chapter 6)

As Table B4 shows, the gift giving patterns reported by condom users and non-users were slightly skewed in opposite directions, although they did not follow perfect curves and although the inner three points of these curves (often, sometimes, rarely) were quite similar.

5. How Men Show Love (Chapter 6)

In the final version of the questionnaire, partnered women were asked how their partners showed them love. Eight condom users and thirty-one non-users provided information. The question was open-ended and during the coding phase it was found that answers fell easily into four categories: partners showed love by meeting either emotional, material, sexual, or other needs. Emotional needs were most frequently met, followed closely by material needs, with sexual needs running a distant third (three women [7.7%, N = 39] mentioned having their sexual needs met).

TABLE B4. Frequency of Gift Offerings Received and Condom Use

	Users (N=154 total answers)	Non-users (N=379 total answers)
Very often	26 (16.9%)	104 (27.4%)
Often	32 (20.8%)	76 (20.1%)
Sometimes	28 (18.2%)	88 (23.2%)
Rarely	10 (7%)	32 (8.4%)
Never	58 (37.7%)	79 (20.8%)

TABLE B5. Condom Use and Women's Views of How Partners Show Love

Meeting women's needs	Users (N=8)	Non-users (N=31)
Emotional needs	4 (50%)	10 (32.3%)
Material needs	1 (12.5%)	11 (35.5%)
Sexual needs	1 (12.5%)	2 (6.5%)
Other needs	2 (25%)	8 (25.8%)

When women's answers were examined in light of their condom-use habits, possibly important differences emerged. As Table B5 shows, four (half) of the condom users wrote that their partners demonstrated love by meeting their emotional needs, while one wrote about her partner showing his love by meeting her material needs. The thirty-one non-users were more evenly split and meeting material needs was a more popular method of showing love: eleven (35.5%) wrote of having material needs met. Ten (32.3%) wrote of having emotional needs met as symbolic of a partner's love.

6. HIV-Testing Desires (Chapter 8)

Thirty-six (40%) of the ninety questionnaire respondents had no desire to be tested for HIV. Sixteen (45.7%) of the thirty-five women who gave reasons for not testing specified that they did not need testing because they trusted their partners; twelve (34.3%) said that they did not want the test because they were not at risk. Seven (20%) of the women uninterested in testing simply did not want to know if they were positive.

Twelve (23.1%, N = 52; data were missing for one woman) of the questionnaire respondents who have been or who want to be tested worried about risks that their partners might be taking; but only seven (13.5%) were certain about these risks. Only one (1.9%) woman got tested because she was taking risks herself. (Note that having thoughts about risk in the context of testing is quite different from having them in general or in the context of sexual intercourse.)

References Cited

Abelove, H.
  1994   "The Politics of the 'Gay Plague': AIDS as a U.S. Ideology." In M.
          Ryan and A. Gordon, eds., *Body Politics: Disease, Desire, and the Family.*
          San Francisco: Westview Press, pp. 3–17.
Abramson, P.
  1992   "Sex, Lies, and Ethnography." In G. Herdt and S. Lindenbaum,
          eds., *The Time of AIDS: Social Analysis, Theory, and Method.* Newbury
          Park, CA: Sage Publications, pp. 101–123.
Advocate
  1993   "Medical Briefs." (11/02). 641:33.
AIDS Alert
  1993   "Research Gaining Support for Vaginal Microbicide." 8(9):134.
Ajzen, I. and M. Fishbein
  1980   *Understanding Attitudes and Predicting Social Behavior.* Englewood
          Cliffs, NJ: Prentice-Hall.
Altman, L.
  1993   "New Strategy Backed for Fighting AIDS." *New York Times,* Nov. 2,
          p. C1.
Amass, L., W. Bickel, S. Higgins, A. Budney, and F. Foerg
  1993   "The Taking of Free Condoms in a Drug Abuse Treatment Clinic:
          The Effects of Location and Posters." *American Journal of Public
          Health* 83(10):1466.
Anderson, E.
  1990   *Streetwise: Race, Class, and Change in an Urban Neighborhood.* Chicago:
          University of Chicago Press.
Anderson, J., A. Hardy, K. Cahill, and S. Aral
  1992   "HIV Antibody Testing and Posttest Counseling in the United
          States: Data from the 1989 National Health Interview Survey."
          American Journal of Public Health 82(11):1533–1535.
Arras, J.
  1990   "AIDS and Reproductive Decisions: Having Children in Fear and
          Trembling." *Milbank Quarterly* 68(3):353–382.
Bailey, F. G.
  1971   "Gifts and Poison." In F. G. Bailey, ed., *Gifts and Poison.* New York:
          Schocken Books, pp. 1–27.

Baltimore Sun
1993   "Women with AIDS Risk Assault by Partners," (10/14) October 14, p. 16A.

Bandura, A.
1989   "Perceived Self-Efficacy in the Exercise of Control over AIDS Infection." In V. Mays, G. Albee, and S. Schneider, eds., *Primary Prevention of AIDS: Psychological Approaches*. Newbury Park, CA: Sage Publications, pp. 128–141.
1977   "Toward a Unifying Theory of Behavioral Change." *Psychological Review* 34:191–215.

Basch, C.
1987   "Focus Group Interview: An Underutilized Research Technique for Improving Theory and Practice in Health Education." *Health Education Quarterly* 14:411–418.

Bates, K.
1990   "AIDS: Is It Genocide?" *Essence* 21:76–78, 116, 118.

Becker, M. and J. Joseph
1988   "AIDS and Behavioral Change to Reduce Risk: A Review." *American Journal of Public Health* 78(4):394–410.

Bender, D. and D. Ewbank
1994   "The Focus Group as a Tool for Health Research: Issues in Design and Analysis." *Health Transition Review* 4(1):63–80.

Bentley, M., G. Pelto, W. Straus, D. Schumann, C. Adegbola, E. de la Pena, G. Oni, K. Brown, and S. Huffman
1988   "Rapid Ethnographic Assessment: Applications in a Diarrhea Management Program." *Social Science and Medicine* 27(1):107–116.

Berrios, D. C., N. Hearst, T. J. Coates, R. Stall, E. S. Hudes, H. Turner, R. Eversley, J. Catania
1993   "HIV Antibody Testing Among Those at Risk for Infection: The National AIDS Behavioral Surveys." *Journal of the American Medical Association* 270(13):1576–1580.

Bezemer, W.
1992   "Women and HIV." *Journal of Psychology and Human Sexuality* 5(1,2):31–36.

Bledsoe, C.
1990   "The Politics of AIDS, Condoms, and Heterosexual Relations in Africa: Recent Evidence from the Local Print Media." In W. Penn Handwerker, ed., *Births and Power: Social Change and the Politics of Reproduction*. San Francisco: Westview Press, pp. 197–223.

Bletzer, K.
1993   "Migrant HIV Education in the Wake of the AIDS Crisis." *Practicing Anthropology* 15(4):13–16.

Bolton, R.
1992   "AIDS and Promiscuity: Muddles in the Models." In R. Bolton and M. Singer, eds., *Rethinking AIDS Prevention*. New York: Gordon and Breach, pp. 7–85.

Bolton, R. and M. Singer
1992   "Introduction. Rethinking HIV Prevention: Critical Assessments of the Content and Delivery of AIDS Risk-Reduction Messages." In R. Bolton and M. Singer eds., *Rethinking AIDS Prevention*. New York: Gordon and Breach, pp. 1–5.

Bor, R., R. Miller, and H. Salt
    1991   "Uptake of HIV Testing Following Counseling." *Sexual and Marital Therapy* 6(1):25–28.
Borden, W.
    1991   "Beneficial Outcomes in Adjustment to HIV Seropositivity." *Social Service Review* 65(3):434–449.
Bott, E.
    1971   *Family and Social Network: Roles, Norms, and External Relationships in*
    [1957]   *Ordinary Urban Families* 2nd edition, New York: Free Press.
Bower, B.
    1991   "Risky Sex and AIDS." *Science News* 140(9)(8/31):141.
Boyd, K. (on behalf of the Institute of Medical Ethics Working Party)
    1990   "HIV Infection: The Ethics of Anonymised Testing and of Testing Pregnant Women." *Journal of Medical Ethics* 16:173–178.
Browner, C.
    1983   "Male Pregnancy Symptoms in Urban Colombia." *American Ethnologist* 10(3):494–511.
Bruhn, J. and B. Philips
    1984   "Measuring Social Support: A Synthesis of Current Approaches." *Journal of Behavioral Medicine* 7(2):151–169.
Campbell, C.
    1990   "Women and AIDS." *Social Science and Medicine* 30(4):407–15.
Cancellieri, F., J. Fine, S. Holman, A. Sutherland, S. Landesman, and B. Bihari
    1988   "Psychological Reactions to HIV-Spectrum Disease: A Comparison of Responses." In R. Schinazi and A. Nahmias, eds., *AIDS in Children, Adolescents and Heterosexual Adults.* New York: Elsevier, pp. 207–210.
Carovano, K.
    1991   "More Than Mothers and Whores: Redefining the AIDS Prevention Needs of Women." *International Journal of Health Services* 21(1): 131–142.
Cary, L.
    1992   "Why It's Not Just Paranoia: An American History of 'Plans' for Blacks." *Newsweek,* 6 April, p. 23.
Catania, J., T. Coates, S. Kegeles, M. Fullilove, J. Peterson, B. Marin, D. Siegel, and S. Hulley
    1992   "Condom Use in Multi-Ethnic Neighborhoods of San Francisco: The Population-Based AMEN (AIDS in Multi-Ethnic Neighborhoods) Study." *American Journal of Public Health* 82(2):284–287.
Catania, J., T. Coates, J. Peterson, M. Dolcini, S. Kegeles, D. Siegel, E. Golden, and M. Fullilove
    1993   "Changes in Condom Use Among Black, Hispanic, and White Heterosexuals in San Francisco: The AMEN Cohort Survey." *Journal of Sex Research* 30(2):121–128.
Catania, J., S. Kegeles, and T. Coates
    1990   "Towards an Understanding of Risk Behavior: An AIDS Risk Reduction" Model (AARM). *Health Education Quarterly* 17(1):53–72.
CDC [Centers for Disease Control and Prevention]
    1994a   *HIV/AIDS Surveillance Report* 5(4).
    1994b   "Zidovudine for the Prevention of HIV Transmission from Mother to Infant." *Morbidity and Mortality Weekly Report* 43(16):285–287.

1993a   *HIV/AIDS Prevention* 4(2).
1993b   *HIV/AIDS Surveillance Report* 5(1).
1993c   *HIV/AIDS Surveillance Report* 5(2).
1993d   "Update: Mortality Attributable to HIV Infection/AIDS Among Persons Aged 25–44 Years—United States, 1990 and 1991." *Morbidity and Mortality Weekly Report* 42(25):481–486.
1990   "Estimates of HIV Prevalence and Projected AIDS Cases: Summary of a Workshop, October 31–November 1, 1989." *Morbidity and Mortality Weekly Report* 39(7):110–119.
CDC National AIDS Clearinghouse
1993   Soviets Secretly Tried to Blame U.S. for AIDS—CIA (Reuters 9/30/93). Information, Inc., Bethesda, MD.
1995   "Facts About . . . Women and AIDS." *Fact Sheet,* February 9. Rockville, MD.
Chiodo, G. and S. Tolle
1992   "A Challenge to Doctor-Patient Confidentiality: When HIV-Positive Patients Refuse Disclosure to Spouses." *Dental Ethics* 40(4):275–277.
Cleary, P., N. Van Devanter, T. Rogers, E. Singer, R. Shipton-Levy, F. Steilen, A. Stuart, J. Avorn, and J. Pindyck
1991   "Behavior Changes After Notification of HIV Infection." *American Journal of Public Health* 81(12):1586–1590.
Cline, R., K. Freeman, and S. Johnson
1990   "Talk Among Sexual Partners About AIDS: Factors Differentiating Those Who Talk From Those Who Do Not." *Communication Research* 17(6):792–808.
Coates, T., R. Stall, S. Kegeles, B. Lo, S. Morin, and L. McKusick
1988   "AIDS Antibody Testing: Will It Stop the AIDS Epidemic? Will It Help People Infected With HIV?" *American Psychologist* 11:859–864.
Cochran, S.
1991   "Psychosocial HIV Interventions in the Second Decade: A Note on Social Support and Social Networks." *Counseling Psychologist* 19(4):551–557.
1989   "Women and HIV Infection: Issues in Prevention and Behavioral Change." In V. Mays, G. Albee, and S. Schneider, eds., *Primary Prevention of AIDS: Psychological Approaches.* Newbury Park, CA: Sage Publications, pp. 309–327.
Cochran, S. and V. Mays
1991   "Psychosocial HIV Interventions in the Second Decade: A Note on Social Support and Social Networks." *Counseling Psychologist* 19(4):551–557.
Copelon, R.
1990   "From Privacy to Autonomy: The Conditions for Sexual and Reproductive Freedom." In M. G. Fried, ed., *From Abortion to Reproductive Freedom: Transforming a Movement.* Boston: South End Press, pp. 27–43.
Corea, G.
1992   *The Invisible Epidemic: The Story of Women and AIDS.* New York: HarperCollins.
Coyle, S., R. Boruch, and C. Turner, eds.
1991   *Evaluating AIDS Prevention Programs.* Expanded edition. Washington, DC: National Academy Press.

Cullen, B.
1991   "Human Immunodeficiency Virus as a Prototypic Complex Retro-
virus." *Journal of Virology* 65(3):1053–1056.

CUPSC [Center for Urban Poverty and Social Change]
1992   *Neighborhood Profiles: A Profile of Social and Economic Conditions in the
City of Cleveland.* Vol. II. Cleveland: Center for Urban Poverty and
Social Change, Mandel School of Applied Social Sciences, Case
Western Reserve University.

Curtis, T.
1992   "The Origin of AIDS." *Rolling Stone,* 19 March, pp. 54–108.

Dalton, H.
1989   "AIDS in Blackface." *Daedalus* 118(3):205–227.

De Bruyn, M.
1992   "Women and AIDS in Developing Countries." *Social Science and
Medicine* 34(3):249–262.

De La Cancela, V.
1989   "Minority AIDS Prevention: Moving Beyond Cultural Perspectives
Towards Sociopolitical Empowerment." *AIDS Education and Prevention* 1(2):141–153.

DeParle, J.
1990   "Talk of Government Being Out to Get Blacks Falls on More Atten-
tive Ears." *New York Times,* Oct. 29, p. B7.

DiClemente, R.
1992   "Psychosocial Determinants of Condom Use Among Adolescents."
In R. DiClemente, ed., *Adolescents and AIDS: A Generation in Jeopardy.*
Newbury Park, CA: Sage Publications, pp. 34–51.

Doll, L., P. O'Malley, A. Pershing, W. Darrow, N. Hessol, and A. Lifson
1990   "High-Risk Sexual Behavior and Knowledge of HIV Antibody Status in the San Francisco City Clinic Cohort." *Health Psychology*
9(3):253–265.

Dorfman, L., P. Derish, and J. Cohen
1992   "Hey Girlfriend: An Evaluation of Aids Prevention Among Women
in the Sex Industry." *Health Education Quarterly* 19(1):25–40.

Dressler, W.
1991   *Stress and Adaptation in the Context of Culture.* Albany: State University
of New York Press.

Dunbar, S. and S. Rehm
1992   "On Visibility: AIDS, Deception by Patients, and the Responsibility
of the Doctor." *Journal of Medical Ethics* 18:180–185.

Earl, W., C. Martindale, and D. Cohn
1991–92 "Adjustment: Denial in the Styles of Coping with HIV Infection."
Omega 24(1):35–47.

Edgar, H.
1992   "Outside the Community." *Hastings Center Report* 22(6):32–35.

Evans-Pritchard, E. E.
1968   *The Nuer: A Description of the Modes of Livelihood and Political Institu-
tions of a Nilotic People.* New York: Oxford University Press.

Farmer, P.
1992   *AIDS and Accusation: Haiti and the Geography of Blame.* Berkeley: University of California Press.

Farmer, P. and J. Y. Kim
  1991   "Anthropology, Accountability, and the Prevention of AIDS." *Journal of Sex Research* 28(2):203–221.
Fischoff, B., S. Lichtenstein, P. Slovic, S. L. Derby, and R. L. Keeny
  1981   *Acceptable Risk.* New York: Cambridge University Press.
Fishbein, M. and S. Middlestadt
  1989   "Using the Theory of Reasoned Action as a Framework for Understanding and Changing AIDS-Related Behaviors." In V. Mays, G. Albee, and S. Schneider, eds., *Primary Prevention of AIDS: Psychological Approaches.* Newbury Park, CA: Sage Publications, pp. 93–110.
Fisher, J.
  1988   "Possible Effects of Reference Group-Based Social Influence on AIDS-Risk Behavior and AIDS Prevention." *American Psychologist* 43(11):914–920.
Flaskerud, J. and C. Rush
  1989   "AIDS and Traditional Health Beliefs and Practices of Black Women." *Nursing Research* 38(4):210–215.
Freeman, H.
  1991   "HIV Testing of Asymptomatic Patients in U.S. Hospitals." *Medical Care* 28(2):87–96.
Freilich, M.
  1968   "Sex, Secrets, and Systems." In S. Gerber ed., *The Family in the Caribbean.* San Juan, PR: Institute of Caribbean Studies, pp. 47–62.
Fullilove, M., R. Fullilove III, K. Haynes, and S. Gross
  1990   "Black Women and AIDS Prevention: A View Towards Understanding the Gender Rules." *Journal of Sex Research* 27(1):47–64.
Gard, L.
  1990   "Patient Disclosure of Human Immunodeficiency Virus (HIV) Status to Parents: Clinical Considerations." *Professional Psychology: Research and Practice* 21(4):252–256.
Gardner, W.
  1993   "A Life-Span Rational-Choice Theory of Risk Taking." In N. Bell and R. Bell, eds., *Adolescent Risk Taking.* Newbury Park, CA: Sage Publications, pp. 66–83.
Gerbert, B., J. Sumser, and B. T. Maguire
  1991   "The Impact of Who You Know and Where You Live on Opinions About AIDS and Health Care." *Social Science and Medicine* 32(6): 677–681.
Geringer, W., S. Marks, W. Allen, and K. Armstrong
  1993   "Knowledge, Attitudes, and Behavior Related to Condom Use and STDs in a High Risk Population." *Journal of Sex Research* 30(1):75–83.
Giesecke, J., K. Ramstedt, F. Granath, T. Ripa, G. Rado, and M. Westrell
  1991   "Efficacy of Partner Notification for HIV Infection." *Lancet* 338(8775):1096–1099.
Gladwell, M.
  1992   "The Message on Safe Sex Just Isn't Getting Through and the Experts Aren't Sure What to Do Next. *Washington Post* National Weekly Edition, May 25–31, p. 38.
Glick Schiller, N.
  1993   "The Invisible Women: Caregiving and the Construction of AIDS Health Services." *Culture, Medicine, and Psychiatry* 17(4):431–454.

1992   "What's Wrong with This Picture: The Hegemonic Construction of Culture in AIDS Research in the United States." *Medical Anthropology Quarterly* N.S. 6(3):237–254.

Green, J.
1989   "Post-test Counselling." In J. Green and A. McCreaner, eds., *Counselling in HIV Infection and AIDS*. Boston: Blackwell Scientific Publications, 28–68.

Guinan, M.
1993   "Black Communities' Belief in 'AIDS as Genocide': A Barrier to Overcome for HIV Prevention." *Annals of Epidemiology* 3(2):193–195.

Gupta, G. and E. Weiss
1993   "Women's Lives and Sex: Implications for AIDS Prevention." *Culture, Medicine and Psychiatry* 17(4):399–412.

Handwerker, W. P.
1993   "Gender Power Differences May be STD Risk Factors for the Next Generation. *Journal of Women's Health* 2:301–316.

Hansen, W., G. Hahn, and B. Wolkenstein
1990   "Perceived Personal Immunity: Beliefs About Susceptibility to AIDS." *Journal of Sex Research* 27(4):622–628.

Hardy, A. and A. Biddlecom
1991   AIDS Knowledge and Attitudes of Black Americans: United States, 1990: Provisional Data From the National Health Interview Survey. Advance data from *Vital and Health Statistics*, No. 206. Hyattsville, MD: National Center for Health Statistics.

Harrison, D., K. Wambach, J. Byers, A. Imershein, P. Levine, K. Maddox, D. Quadagno, M. Fordyce, and M. Jones
1991   "AIDS Knowledge and Risk Behaviors Among Culturally Diverse Women." *AIDS Education and Prevention* 3(2):79–89.

Hays, R., L. McKusick, L. Pollack, R. Hillard, C. Hoff, and T. Coates
1993   "Disclosing HIV Seropositivity to Significant Others." *AIDS* 7(3):425–431.

Henry, K., M. Maki, K. Willenbring, and S. Campbell
1991   "The Impact of Experience with AIDS on HIV Testing and Counseling Practices: A Study of U.S. Infectious Disease Teaching Hospitals and Minnesota Hospitals." *AIDS Education and Prevention* 3(4):313–321.

Herdt, G. and A. Boxer
1991   "Ethnographic Issues in the Study of AIDS." *Journal of Sex Research* 28(2):171–187.

Herek, G., and J. Capitanio
1994   "Conspiracies, Contagion, and Compassion: Trust and Public Reactions to AIDS." *AIDS Education and Prevention* 6(4):365–375.

Holtgrave, D., R. Valdiserri, A. Gerber, and A. Hinman
1993   "Human Immunodeficiency Virus Counseling, Testing, Referral, and Partner Notification Services." *Archives of Internal Medicine* 153:1225–1230.

House, W., A. Faulk, and M. Kubovchik
1990   "Sexual Behavior of Inner-City Women." *Journal of Sex Education and Therapy* 16(3):172–184.

Hutchinson, J.
1993   "Delayed Diagnosis of HIV/AIDS Among Women in the United States: Its Causes and Health Repercussions." Ms. in files of the author.

Ingstad, B.
1990   "The Cultural Construction of AIDS and Its Consequences for Prevention in Botswana." *Medical Anthropology Quarterly* 4(1):28–40.

Institute of Medicine (U.S.A.)
1988   *Confronting AIDS: Update 1988.* Washington, DC: National Academy Press.

Irwin, C.
1993   "Adolescence and Risk Taking: How Are They Related?" In N. Bell and R. Bell, eds., *Adolescent Risk Taking.* Newbury Park, CA: Sage Publications, pp. 7–28.

JAMA (*Journal of the American Medical Association*)
1993   "Update: Acquired Immunodeficiency Syndrome — United States, 1992." 270(8):930–931. Published originally in *Morbidity and Mortality Weekly Report* 42(1993):551–557.

Janz, N. and M. Becker
1984   "The Health Belief Model: A Decade Later." *Health Education Quarterly* 11(1):1–47.

Jemmott, L. and J. Jemmott
1991   "Applying the Theory of Reasoned Action to AIDS Risk Behavior: Condom Use Among Black Women." *Nursing Research* 40(4):228–234.

Johnson, E.
1993   *Risky Sexual Behaviors Among African-Americans.* Westport, CT: Praeger Publishers.

Jones, J.
1992   "The Tuskegee Legacy: AIDS and the Black Community." *Hastings Center Report* 22(6):38–40.

Jones, R.
1991   "The Political and Economic Dynamics of STDs." Paper presented at the 90th Annual Meeting of the American Anthropological Association, Chicago.

Joseph, J., R. Kessler, C. Wortman, J. Kirscht, M. Tal, S. Caumartin, S. Eshleman, and M. Eller
1989   "Are There Psychological Costs Associated with Changes in Behavior to Reduce AIDS Risk?" In V. Mays, G. Albee, and S. Schneider, eds., *Primary Prevention of AIDS: Psychological Approaches.* Newbury Park, CA: Sage Publications, pp. 209–224.

Kammerer, C. and P. Symonds
1992   "Hill Tribes Endangered at Thailand's Periphery." *Cultural Survival Quarterly* 16(3):23–25.

Kane, S. and T. Mason
1992   " 'IV Drug Users' and 'Sex Partners': The Limits of Epidemiological Categories and the Ethnography of Risk." In G. Herdt and S. Lindenbaum, eds., *The Time of AIDS: Social Analysis, Theory, and Method.* Newbury Park, CA: Sage Publications, pp. 199–222.

Kegeles, S., N. Adler, and C. Irwin
1988   "Sexually Active Adolescents and Condoms: Changes over One

Year in Knowledge, Attitudes and Use." *American Journal of Public Health* 78:460–467.

Kegeles, S., J. Catania, and T. Coates
1988   "Intentions to Communicate Positive HIV-Antibody Status to Sex Partners." *Journal of American Medical Association* 259:216–217.

Kelly, J., J. St. Lawrence, H. Hood, and T. Brasfield
1989   "Behavioral Intervention to Reduce AIDS Risk Activities." *Journal of Consulting and Clinical Psychology* 57(1):60–67.

Kilbride, P. and J. C. Kilbride
1990   *Changing Family Life in East Africa: Women and Children at Risk.* University Park: Pennsylvania State University Press.

Kimmel, A. and R. Keefer
1991   "Psychological Correlates of the Transmission and Acceptance of Rumors About AIDS." *Journal of Applied Psychology* 21(19):1608–1628.

Kinsey, K.
1994   " 'But I Know My Man': HIV/AIDS Risk Appraisals and Heuristical Reasoning Patterns Among Childbearing Women." *Holistic Nurse Practitioner* 8(2):79–88.

Kirscht, J. and J. Joseph
1989   "The Health Belief Model: Some Implications for Behavior Change, with Reference to Homosexual Males." In V. Mays, G. Albee, and S. Schneider, eds., *Primary Prevention of AIDS: Psychological Approaches.* Newbury Park, CA: Sage Publications, pp. 111–127.

Kleinman, A., L. Eisenberg, and B. Good
1978   "Culture, Illness, and Care: Clinical Lessons from Anthropologic and Cross-Cultural Research." *Annals of Internal Medicine* 88:251–258.

Kline, A., E. Kline, and E. Oken
1992   "Minority Women and Sexual Choice in the Age of AIDS." *Social Science and Medicine* 34(4):447–457.

Kline, A. and J. Strickler
1993   "Perceptions of Risk for AIDS Among Women in Drug Treatment." *Health Psychology* 12(4):313–323.

Kline, A. and M. VanLandingham
1994   "HIV-Infected Women and Sexual Risk Reduction: The Relevance of Existing Models of Behavioral Change." *AIDS Education and Prevention* 6(5):390–402.

Kurth, A. and M. Hutchison
1989   "A Context for HIV Testing in Pregnancy." *Journal of Nurse-Midwifery* 34(5):259–265.

Lancet
1991   Partner Notification for Preventing HIV Infection." 338(8775): 1112–1113.

Landis, S., J. Earp, and G. Koch
1992   "Impact of HIV Testing and Counseling on Subsequent Sexual Behavior." *AIDS Education and Prevention* 4(1)61–70.

Landis, S., V. Schoenbach, D. Weber, M. Mittal, B. Krishan, K. Lewis, and G. Koch
1992   "Results of a Randomized Trial of Partner Notification in Cases of HIV Infection in North Carolina." *New England Journal of Medicine* 326(2):101–106.

Lang, N.
   1991   "Stigma, Self-Esteem, and Depression: Psycho-Social Responses to Risk of AIDS." *Human Organization* 50(1):66–72.
Larson, A.
   1989   "Social Context of Human Immunodeficiency Virus Transmission in Africa: Historical and Cultural Bases of East and Central African Sexual Relations." *Reviews of Infectious Diseases* 2(5):716–731.
Laryea, M. and L. Gien
   1993   "The Impact of HIV-Positive Diagnosis on the Individual, Part 1: Stigma, Rejection, and Loneliness." *Clinical Nursing Research* 2(3): 245–266.
Lazarus, E.
   1990   "Falling Through the Cracks: Contradictions and Barriers to Care in a Prenatal Clinic." *Medical Anthropology* 12:269–287.
Leap, W. and K. O'Connor
   1993   "Introduction: Applying Anthropology in HIV/AIDS Research." *Practicing Anthropology* 15(4):3–4.
Lester, C. and L. Saxxon
   1988   "AIDS in the Black Community: The Plague, the Politics, the People." *Death Studies* 12:563–571.
Leventhal, H., D. Meyer, and D. Nerenz
   1977   "The Common Sense Representation of Illness Danger." In S. Rachman, ed., *Contributions to Medical Psychology*. New York: Pergamon Press, pp. 7–30.
Levine, C. and N. Dubler
   1990   "Uncertain Risks and Bitter Realities: The Reproductive Choices of HIV-Infected Women." *Milbank Quarterly* 68(3):321–351.
Lewis, D. and J. Watters
   1989   "Human Immunodeficiency Virus Seroprevalence in Female Intravenous Drug Users: The Puzzle of Black Women's Risk." *Social Science and Medicine* 29(9):1071–1076.
Liebow, E.
   1967   *Tally's Corner: a Study of Negro Streetcorner Men*. Boston: Little, Brown and Company.
Limandri, B.
   1989   "Disclosure of Stigmatizing Conditions: The Discloser's Perspective." *Archives of Psychiatric Nursing* 3(2):69–78.
Linden, C., S. Kegeles, N. Hearst, P. Grant, and D. Johnson
   1990   "Heterosexual Behaviors and Factors that Influence Condom Use Among Patients Attending a Sexually Transmitted Disease Clinic - San Francisco." *Morbidity and Mortality Weekly Report* 39:685–689.
Lindsay, M., H. Peterson, E. Taylor, M. Blunt, S. Willis, and L. Klein
   1990   "Routine Human Immunodeficiency Virus Infection Screening of Women Requesting Induced First-Trimester Abortion in an Inner-City Population." *Obstetrics and Gynecology* 76(3):347–350.
Lindsay, M., H. Peterson, T. Feng, B. Slade, S. Willis, and L. Klein
   1989   "Routine Antepartum Human Immunodeficiency Virus Infection Screening in an Inner-City Population." *Obstetrics and Gynecology* 74(3):289–294.
Mann, J., D. Tarantola, and T. Neter, eds.
   1992   *AIDS in the World*. Cambridge, MA: Harvard University Press.

Mantell, J., S. Tross, B. Rapkin, B. Ortiz-Torres, K. Anastos, C. Ramis, and M. Arnouk
    1992   "Determinants of the Decision to Seek HIV Testing Among Inner-City Women." Presented at the Eighth International Conference on AIDS, Amsterdam, July; Poster Session #POC4826.

Marks, G., J. Richardson, and N. Maldonado
    1991   "Self-Disclosure of HIV Infection to Sexual Partners." *American Journal of Public Health* 81(10):1321–1322.

Marks, G., J. Richardson, M. Ruiz, and N. Maldonado
    1992a   "HIV-Infected Men's Practices in Notifying Past Sexual Partners of Infection Risk." *Public Health Reports* 107(1):100–106.

Marks, G., N. Bundek, J. Richardson, M. Ruiz, N. Maldonado, and H. Mason
    1992b   "Self-Disclosure of HIV Infection: Preliminary Results from a Sample of Hispanic Men." *Health Psychology* 11(5):300–306.

Massey, D. and N. Denton
    1988   "Suburbanization and Segregation in U.S. Metropolitan Areas." *American Journal of Sociology* 94(3):592–626.

Maticka-Tyndale, E.
    1992   "Social Construction of HIV Transmission and Prevention Among Heterosexual Young Adults." *Social Problems* 39:230–252.

Mauss, M.
    1967   *The Gift.* New York: Norton.

Mays, V.
    1989   "AIDS Prevention in Black Populations: Prevention of a Safer Kind." In V. Mays, G. Albee, and S. Schneider, eds., *Primary Prevention of AIDS: Psychological Approaches.* Newbury Park, CA: Sage Publications, pp. 264–279.

Mays, V. and S. Cochran
    1990   "Methodological Issues in the Assessment and Prediction of AIDS Risk-Related Sexual Behaviors Among Black Americans." In B. Voeller, J. Reinisch, and M. Gottlieb, eds., *AIDS and Sex.* New York: Oxford University Press, pp. 97–120.
    1988   "Issues in the Perception of AIDS Risk and Risk Reduction Activities by Black and Hispanic/Latina Women." *American Psychologist* 43(11):949–957.
    1987   "Acquired Immunodeficiency Syndrome and Black Americans: Special Psychosocial Issues." *Public Health Reports* 102(2):224–231.

McCann, K. and E. Wadsworth
    1991   "The Experience of Having a Positive HIV Antibody Test." *AIDS Care* 3(1):43–53.

McCain, N. and L. Gramling
    1992   "Living with Dying: Coping with HIV Disease." *Issues in Mental Health Nursing* 13:271–284.

McCusker, J., A. Stoddard, and E. McCarthy
    1992   "The Validity of Self-reported HIV Antibody Test Results." *American Journal of Public Health* 82(4):567–569.

McDonald, M., J. Hamilton, and D. Durack
    1983   "Hepatitis B Surface Antigen Could Harbour the Infective Agent of AIDS." *Lancet* 2(8355):882–884.

McGarrahan, P.
    1994   *Transcending AIDS: Nurses and HIV Patients in New York City.* Philadelphia: University of Pennsylvania Press.

McKeganey, N. and M. Barnard
1992   *AIDS, Drugs and Sexual Risk: Lives in the Balance*. Philadelphia: Open University Press.

McKusick, L., T. Coates, J. Wiley, S. Morin, and R. Stall
1984   "Prevention of HIV Infection Among Gay and Bisexual Men: Two Longitudinal Studies." Paper presented at the Third International Conference on AIDS, Washington, D.C.

McQuillan, G., Khare, M., Ezzati-Rice, T., Karon, J., Schable, C. and R. Murphy
1994   "The Seroepidemiology of Human Immunodeficiency Virus in the United States Household Population: NHANES III, 1988–1991." *Journal of Acquired Immune Deficiency Syndrome* 7(11):1195–1201.

Meadows, J., S. Jenkinson, J. Catalan, and B. Gazzard
1990   "Voluntary HIV Testing in the Antenatal Clinic: Differing Uptake Rates for Individual Counselling Midwives." *AIDS Care* 2(3)229–233.

Medalie, J., G. Kitson, and S. Zyzanski
1981   "A Family Epidemiological Model: A Practice and Research Concept for Family Medicine." *Journal of Family Practice* 12(1):79–87.

Metts, S. and M. Fitzpatrick
1992   "Thinking About Safer Sex: The Risky Business of 'Know Your Partner' Advice." In T. Edgar, M. Fitzpatrick, V. Freimuth, eds., *AIDS: A Communication Perspective*. Hillsdale, NJ: Lawrence Earlbaum Associates, p. 1–19.

Miller, H., C. Turner, and L. Moses, eds.
1990   *AIDS: The Second Decade*. Washington, DC: National Academy Press.

Millstein, S.
1993   "Perceptual, Attributional, and Affective Processes in Perceptions of Vulnerability Through the Life Span." In N. Bell and R. Bell, eds., *Adolescent Risk Taking*. Newbury Park, CA: Sage Publications, pp. 55–65.

Moore, R., D. Stanton, R. Gopalan, and R. Chaisson
1994   "Racial Differences in the Use of Drug Therapy for HIV Disease in an Urban Community." *New England Journal of Medicine* 330:763–768.

Muir, M.
1991   *The Environmental Context of AIDS*. New York: Praeger Publishers.

Nation's Health
1993   "APHA Fights Criminalization of HIV Exposure in Illinois Court." 23(10):9.

New York Times
1992   "The AIDS 'Plot' Against Blacks." May 12, p. A14.
1993   "U.N. Agency Reports AIDS Virus Spreading Very Quickly in Africa." December 13, p. B8.

Nichols, M.
1990   "Women and Acquired Immunodeficiency Syndrome: Issues for Prevention." In B. Voeller, J. Reinisch, and M. Gottlieb, eds., *AIDS and Sex: An Integrated Biomedical and Biobehavioral Approach*. New York: Oxford University Press, pp. 375–392.

NMHDU (*New Mexico HIV Disease Update*)
1994   "861 AIDS Cases Reported by 12/31/93." (Winter)

Nyamathi, A., P. Shuler, and M. Porche
1990   "AIDS Educational Program for Minority Women at Risk." *Family and Community Health* 13(2):54–64.

O'Campo, P., M. de Boer, R. Faden, A. Gielen, N. Kass, and R. Chaisson
1992   "Discrepancies Between Women's Personal Interview Data and Medical Record Documentation of Illicit Drug Use, Sexually Transmitted Diseases, and HIV Infection." *Medical Care* 30(10):965–971.

Oliver, W.
1989   "Sexual Conquest and Patterns of Black-on-Black Violence: A Structural-Cultural Perspective." *Violence and Victims* 4(4):257–273.

Onorato, I., M. Gwinn, and T. Dondero
1994   "Applications of Data from the CDC Family of Surveys." *Public Health Reports* 109(2):204–211.

Orr, S., D. Celentano, J. Santelli, and L. Burwell
1994   "Depressive Symptoms and Risk Factors for HIV Acquisition Among Black Women Attending Urban Health Centers in Baltimore. *AIDS Education and Prevention* 6(3):230–246.

Orth-Gomer, K. and A. Unden
1987   "The Measurement of Social Support in Population Surveys." *Social Science and Medicine* 24(1):83–94.

Ostrow, D., J. Jill, A. Nonjan, R. Kessler, C. Emmons, J. Phair, R. Fox, L. Kingsley, J. Dudley, J. Chmiel, and M. Kanraden
1986   "Psychosocial Aspects of AIDS Risk." *Psychopharmacology Bulletin* 22:678–683.

Pappaioanou, M., J. George, W. Hannon, M. Gwinn, T. Dandero, G. Grady, R. Hoff, A. Willoughby, A. Wright, A. Novello, and J. Curran
1990   "HIV Seroprevalence Surveys of Childbearing Women — Objectives, Methods, and Uses of the Data. *Public Health Reports* 105(2): 147–152.

Pelto, P. and G. Pelto
1990   "Methods in Medical Anthropology." In T. Johnson and C. Sargent, eds., *Medical Anthropology: Contemporary Theory and Method.* New York: Praeger Publishers, pp. 269–297.

Perloff, L. and B. Fetzer
1986   "Self-Other Judgments and Perceived Vulnerability to Victimization." *Journal of Personality and Social Psychology* 50(3):502–510.

Perry, S., C. Card, M. Moffatt, T. Ashman, B. Fishman, and L. Jacobsberg
1994   "Self-Disclosure of HIV Infection to Sexual Partners After Repeated Counseling." *AIDS Education and Prevention* 6(5):403–411.

Perry, S., J. Ryan, K. Fogel, B. Fishman, and L. Jacobsberg
1990   "Voluntarily Informing Others of Positive HIV Test Results: Patterns of Notification by Infected Gay Men." *Hospital and Community Psychiatry* 41(5):549–551.

Pinkerton, M. and P. Abramson
1992   "Is Risky Sex Rational?" *Journal of Sex Research* 29(4):561–568.

Pittman, K., P. Wilson, S. Adams-Taylor, and S. Randolph
1992   "Making Sexuality Education and Prevention Programs Relevant for African-American Youth." *Journal of School Health* 62(7):339–344.

Pivnick, A.
1993   "HIV Infection and the Meaning of Condoms." *Culture, Medicine, and Psychiatry* 17(4):431–453.

Pivnick, A., A. Jacobson, K. Eric, M. Mulvihill, M. Hsu, and E. Drucker
1991   Reproductive Decisions Among HIV-Infected, Drug-Using Women: The Importance of Mother-Child Coresidence." *Medical Anthropology Quarterly* N.S. 5(2):153–169.

Prohaska, T., G. Albrecht, J. Levy, N. Sugrue, and K. Joung-Hwa
1990   Determinants of Self-Perceived Risk for AIDS. *Journal of Health and Social Behavior* 31:384–394.

Quimby, E.
1992   "Anthropological Witnessing for African-Americans: Power, Responsibility, and Choice in the Age of AIDS." In G. Herdt and S. Lindenbaum, eds., *The Time of AIDS: Social Analysis, Theory, and Method*. Newbury Park, CA: Sage Publications, pp. 159–184.

Quirk, K.
1993   "Ethnography and Outreach: The Benefits of Team Research." *Practicing Anthropology* 15(4):41–43.

Rensberger, B.
1993   "Teenage Girls Are on the 'Leading Edge' of the AIDS Scourge." *Washington Post* (National Weekly Edition), Aug. 9–15, p. 34.

Rolling Stone
1993   " 'Origin of AIDS' Update." 9 December, p. 38.

Rosen, D. and W. Blank
1992   "Women and HIV." In H. Land, ed., *AIDS: A Complete Guide to Psychosocial Intervention*. Milwaukee, WI: Family Service America.

Rubin, L.
1976   *Worlds of Pain: Life in the Working-Class Family*. New York: Basic Books.

Rushforth, S.
1994   "Political Resistance in a Contemporary Hunter-Gatherer Society: More About Bearlake Athapaskan Knowledge and Authority." *American Ethnologist* 21(2):335–352.

Schmidt, D.
1978   "The Family as The Unit of Medical Care." *Journal of Family Practice* 7(2):303–313.

Schneider, B.
1988   "Gender and AIDS." In R. Kulstad, ed., *AIDS 1988: AAAS Symposia Papers*. Washington DC: American Association for the Advancement of Science.

Schnell, D., D. Higgins, R. Wilson, G. Goldbaum, D. Cohn, and R. Wolitski
1992   "Men's Disclosure of HIV Test Results to Male Primary Sex Partners." *American Journal of Public Health* 82(12):1675–1676.

Schoenborn, C., S. Marsh, and A. Hardy
1994   "AIDS Knowledge and Attitudes for 1992: Data from the National Health Interview Survey." *Advance Data from Vital and Health Statistics* No. 243. Hyattsville, MD: National Center for Health Statistics.

Schoepf, B., R. wa Nkera, C. Schoepf, W. Engundu, and P. Ntsomo
1988   "AIDS and Society in Central Africa: a View from Zaire." In N. Miller and R. Rockwell, eds., *AIDS in Africa: The Social and Policy Impact*. Lewiston, NY: Edwin Mellen Press, pp. 211–233.

Schwartz, T.
1978   "Where is the Culture? Personality as the Distributive Locus of Culture." In G. Spindler, ed., *The Making of Psychological Anthropology*. Berkeley: University of California Press, pp. 419–441.

Secter, B.
1988   "New Black Attempt to Link AIDS, Jews." *San Francisco Chronicle,* June 10, p. A4.
Seidman, S., W. Mosher, and S. Aral
1992   "Women with Multiple Sexual Partners: United States, 1988." *American Journal of Public Health* 82(10):1388–1394.
Shervington, D.
1993   "The Acceptability of the Female Condom Among Low-Income African-American Women." *Journal of the National Medical Association* 85(5):341–347.
Shtarkshall, R. and T. Awerbuch
1992   "It Takes Two to Tango But One to Infect." *Journal of Sex and Marital Therapy* 18(2):121–127.
Sibthorpe, B.
1992   "The Social Construction of Sexual Relationships as a Determinant of HIV Risk Perception and Condom Use Among Injection Drug Users." *Medical Anthropology Quarterly,* N.S. 6(3):255–270.
Snow L.
1974   "Folk Medical Beliefs and Their Implications for Care of Patients: A Review Based on Studies Among Black Americans." *Annals of Internal Medicine* 81(1):82–96.
Sobo, E. J.
n.d.   "Love, Jealousy, and Unsafe Sex Among Impoverished Inner-City Women." In M. Singer, ed., *The Political Economy of AIDS* (in review).
1995   "Finance, Romance, Social Support, and Condom Use Among Impoverished Inner-City Women." *Human Organization* 54(2):115–128.
1994   "Attitudes Toward HIV Testing Among Inner-City Women." *Medical Anthropology* 16(2):17–38.
1993a   "Inner-city Women and AIDS: The Psycho-Social Benefits of Unsafe Sex." *Culture, Medicine, and Psychiatry* 17(4):455–485.
1993b   *One Blood: The Jamaican Body.* Albany: State University of New York Press.
Solomon, M. and W. DeJong
1989   "Preventing AIDS and Other STDs Through Condom Promotion: A Patient Education Intervention." *American Journal of Public Health* 79(4):453–458.
Spradley, J.
1980   *Participant Observation.* New York: Holt, Rinehart and Winston.
Stack, C.
1974   *All Our Kin: Strategies for Survival in a Black Community.* New York: Harper.
Stall, R., M. Ekstrand, L. Pollack, L. McKusick, and T. Coates
1990   "Relapse from Safer Sex: The Next Challenge for AIDS Prevention Efforts." *Journal of Acquired Immune Deficiency Syndrome* 3:1181–1187.
Steiner, M., C. Piedrahita, L. Glover, and C. Joanis
1993   "Can Condom Users Likely to Experience Condom Failure Be Identified?" *Family Planning Perspectives* 25(5):220–226.

Stepp, L.
  1994   "Selling Safe Sex." *Washington Post,* Jan. 13, p. ʼC5.
Stevens, C., P. Taylor, E. Zang, J. Morrison, E. Harley, S. de Cordoba, C. Bacino, R. Ting, A. Bodner, M. Sarngadharan, R. Gallo, and P. Rubinstein
  1986   "Human T-Cell Lymphotropic Virus Type III Infection in a Cohort of Homosexual Men in New York City." *Journal of the American Medical Association* 255(16):2167–2172.
Strecker, R.
  1986   Letter to the Editor. *Journal of the Royal Society of Medicine* 79:559–560.
Symons, D.
  1993   "How Risky Is Risky Sex?" *Journal of Sex Research* 30(2):188–191.
Tanner, W. and R. Pollack
  1988   "The Effect of Condom Use and Erotic Instructions on Attitudes Toward Condoms." *Journal of Sex Research* 25(4):537–541.
Taylor, C. and D. Lourea
  1992   "HIV Prevention: A Dramaturgical Analysis and Practical Guide to Creating Safer Sex Interventions." In R. Bolton and M. Singer, eds., *Rethinking AIDS Prevention*. New York: Gordon and Breach, pp. 105–146.
Thomas, S. and S. Quinn
  1991   "The Tuskegee Syphilis Study, 1932 to 1972: Implications for HIV Education and AIDS Risk Education Programs in the Black Community." *American Journal of Public Health* 81(11):1498–1505.
Thompson, J., T. Yager, and J. Martin
  1993   "Estimated Condom Failure and Frequency of Condom Use among Gay Men." *American Journal of Public Health* 83(10):1409–1412.
Timberlake, C. and W. Carpenter
  1991   "Sexuality Attitudes of African American Adults." *Urban League Review* 15(1):71–80.
Treichler, P. A.
  1992   "AIDS, HIV, and the Cultural Construction of Reality." In G. Herdt and S. Lindenbaum, eds., *The Time of AIDS: Social Analysis, Theory, and Method*. Newbury Park, CA: Sage Publications, pp. 65–98.
Tunstall, C., S. Kegeles, P. Darney, M. Tervalon, and G. Oliva
  1991   "Women at Risk for Perinatal AIDS Transmission: The San Francisco Perinatal HIV Reduction and Education Demonstration Activities (PHREDA) Project." Paper presented at the 99th Annual Meeting of the American Psychological Association, San Francisco, August 16.
Turner, C., H. Miller, and L. Moses, eds.
  1989   *AIDS: Sexual Behavior and Intravenous Drug Use*. Washington, DC: National Academy Press.
Turner, P.
  1993   *I Heard It Through the Grapevine: Rumor in African-American Culture*. Los Angeles: University of California Press.
Valdiserri, R., V. Arena, D. Proctor, and F. Bonati
  1989   "The Relationship Between Women's Attitudes About Condoms and Their Use: Implications for Condom Promotion Programs." *American Journal of Public Health* 79(4):499–501.

Van Vugt, J., ed.
1994   *AIDS Prevention and Services: Community Based Research.* Westport, CT: Bergin and Garvey.
Vander Linden, C.
1993   "NIMH Prevention Research Helps Women Change AIDS Risk Behavior." *Public Health Reports* 108(3):413.
VanLandingham, M., J. Knodel, C. Saengtienchai, and A. Pramualratana
1994   "Aren't Sexual Issues Supposed to be Sensitive?" *Health Transition Review* 4(1):85–90.
Voeller, B.
1990   "Heterosexual Anal Intercourse: An AIDS Risk Factor." In B. Voeller, J. Reinisch, and M. Gottlieb, eds., *AIDS and Sex: An Integrated Biomedical and Biobehavioral Approach.* New York: Oxford University Press, pp. 276–311.
Walker, R.
1991   *AIDS Today, Tomorrow: An Introduction to the HIV Epidemic in America.* Atlantic Highlands, NJ: Humanities Press International.
Ward, M.
1993a   "A Different Disease: AIDS and Health Care for Women in Poverty." *Culture, Medicine, and Psychiatry* 17(4):413–430.
1993b   "Poor and Positive: Two Contrasting Views from Inside the AIDS Epidemic." *Practicing Anthropology* 15(4):59–61.
1991   "Cupid's Touch: The Lessons of the Family Planning Movement for the AIDS Epidemic." *Journal of Sex Research* 28(2):289–346.
1990   "The Politics of Adolescent Pregnancy: Turf and Teens in Louisiana." In W. P. Handwerker, ed., *Births and Power: Social Change and the Politics of Reproduction.* San Francisco: Westview Press, pp. 147–164.
Weeks, M., M. Singer, and J. Schensul
1993   "Anthropology and Culturally Targeted AIDS Prevention." *Practicing Anthropology* 15(4):17–20.
Weinberg, M. and C. Williams
1988   "Black Sexuality: A Test of Two Theories." *Journal of Sex Research* 25(2):197–218.
Weinstein, N.
1989   "Perceptions of Personal Susceptibility to Harm." In V. Mays, G. Albee, and S. Schneider, eds., *Primary Prevention of AIDS: Psychological Approaches.* Newbury Park, CA: Sage Publications, pp. 142–167.
1987   "Unrealistic Optimism About Susceptibility to Health Problems: Conclusions from a Community-Wide Sample." *Journal of Behavioral Medicine* 10(5):481–500.
1984   "Why It Won't Happen to Me: Perceptions of Risk Factors and Susceptibility." *Health Psychology* 3(5):431–457.
1982   "Unrealistic Optimism About Susceptibility to Health Problems." *Journal of Behavioral Medicine* 5(4):441–460.
Weiss, R.
1994   "Myths of AIDS." *Discover* 15(12):36–42.
WHO [World Health Organization]
1994   *The Current Global Situation of the HIV/AIDS Pandemic.* Global Programme on AIDS report, Geneva, 4 Jan.

Wildavsky, A.
      1988   *Searching for Safety.* New Brunswick, NJ: Transaction Books.
Wilson, P.
      1986   "Black Culture and Sexuality." *Journal of Social Work and Human Sexuality* 4(3):29–46.
Wilson, W.
      1987   *The Truly Disadvantaged.* Chicago: University of Chicago Press.
Wingood, G. and R. DiClemente
      1992   "Cultural, Gender, and Psychosocial Influences on HIV-related Behavior of African-American Female Adolescents: Implications for the Development of Tailored Prevention Programs." *Ethnicity and Disease* 2(4):381–388.
Winkelstein, W., D. Lyman, N. Padian, R. Grant, M. Samuel, J. Wiley, R. Anderson, W. Lang, J. Riggs, and J. Levy
      1987   "Sexual Practices and Risk of Infection by the Human Immunodeficiency Virus: The San Francisco Men's Health Study." *Journal of the American Medical Association* 257:321–325.
Worth, D.
      1990   "Minority Women and AIDS: Culture, Race, and Gender." In D. Feldman, ed., *Cultural Aspects of AIDS.* New York: Praeger Publishers, pp. 111–136.
      1989   "Sexual Decision-Making and AIDS: Why Condom Promotion among Vulnerable Women is Likely to Fail." *Studies in Family Planning* 20(6):297–307.
Wyatt, G. and K. Dunn
      1991   "Examining Predictors of Sex Guilt in Multiethnic Samples of Women." *Archives of Sexual Behavior* 20(5):471–485.
Wyatt, G., S. Peters, and D. Guthrie
      1988   "Kinsey Revisited, Part II: Comparisons of the Sexual Socialization and Sexual Behavior of Black Women Over 33 Years." *Archives of Sexual Behavior* 17(4):289–332.
Wykoff, R., C. Heath, S. Hollis, S. Leonard, C. Quiller, J. Jones, M. Artzrouni, and R. Parker
      1988   "Contact Tracing to Identify Human Immunodeficiency Virus Infection in a Rural Community." *Journal of the American Medical Association* 259(24):3563–3566.
Zimet, G.
      1992   "Attitudes of Teenagers who Know Someone with AIDS." *Psychology Reports* (70)1–2.
Zimet, G., E. Sobo, J. Jackson, T. Zimmerman, J. Mortimer, C. Yanda, and R. Lazebink
      1995   "Sexual Behaviors, Drug Use, and AIDS Knowledge Among Midwestern Runaways." *Youth and Society* 26(4):460–462.
Zola, I.
      1972   "Medicine as an Institution of Social Control." *Sociological Review* 20(4):487–504.

Index

This book was set in Baskerville and Eras typefaces. Baskerville was designed by John Baskerville at his private press in Birmingham, England, in the eighteenth century. The first typeface to depart from oldstyle typeface design, Baskerville has more variation between thick and thin strokes. In an effort to insure that the thick and thin strokes of his typeface reproduced well on paper, John Baskerville developed the first wove paper, the surface of which was much smoother than the laid paper of the time. The development of wove paper was partly responsible for the introduction of typefaces classified as modern, which have even more contrast between thick and thin strokes.

Eras was designed in 1969 by Studio Hollenstein in Paris for the Wagner Typefoundry. A contemporary script-like version of a sans-serif typeface, the letters of Eras have a monotone stroke and are slightly inclined.

Printed on acid-free paper.